Dyslexia in Children

Dyslexia in Children
Multidisciplinary
Perspectives

Edited by
Angela Fawcett, University of Sheffield
Rod Nicolson, University of Sheffield

Harvester Wheatsheaf
New York   London   Toronto   Sydney   Tokyo   Singapore

First published 1994 by
Harvester Wheatsheaf
Campus 400, Maylands Avenue
Hemel Hempstead
Hertfordshire, HP2 7EZ
A division of
Simon & Schuster International Group

© Harvester Wheatsheaf 1994

Printed and bound in Great Britain by
Biddles Ltd, Guildford and King's Lynn

Library of Congress Cataloging-in-Publication Data

Dyslexia in children : multidisciplinary perspectives / edited by
    Angela Fawcett and Rod Nicolson.
        p.   c.m.
    Includes bibliographical references and indexes.
    ISBN 0-7450-1636-7 (pbk)
    1. Dyslexia—Etiology. 2. Dyslexia—Diagnosis.   I. Fawcett,
Angela.   II. Nicolson, Rod.
RJ496.A5D955   1995
618.92′8553—dc20
                                                                94–30250
                                                                CIP

British Library Cataloguing in Publication Data

A catalogue record for this book is available from the
British Library

ISBN 0-7450-1636-7 (pbk)

1   2   3   4   5   98   97   96   95   94

Contents

Dyslexia: A personal view

Angela Fawcett

The reader may well question the inclusion of chapters on motor skills and vision in a book on dyslexia. Surely, dyslexia is simply a literacy problem? So what led us to come up with the unusual concept of presenting chapters on all the skills?

Let me fill you in on the background and explain my reasons for seeing dyslexia as a more diverse and pervasive problem which impinges on every aspect of everyday life.

My original interest in dyslexia was stimulated by the difficulties experienced by my own son, Matthew, who was first diagnosed as dyslexic at the unusually early age of $5\frac{1}{2}$. In Matthew's case, the discrepancy between his intelligence in the top 1 percent and his inability to recognise a single letter was particularly striking. In my search for an explanation for Matthew's difficulties, I had considered (and dismissed) the possibility of dyslexia, because initially I found it difficult to equate what I read of dyslexia as a language-based deficit with my own verbally able child. Rather than showing language difficulties, Matthew was fascinated to the point of obsession with the subtle nuances of meaning in the English language. Nonetheless, when I examined his language more carefully, it was obvious that he experienced some early difficulties in the pronunciation of polysyllabic words, coupled with some confusion over their application. For example, as a small boy of around 5, he had some difficulty in pronouncing elbow and shoulder, producing 'oboe' and 'soldier' as his best attempts. Not only that, he continually mislabelled the two, which led to some confusion when he fell over and hurt himself. Problems such as these suggested an underlying deficit beneath his apparent competence.

Matthew needed to be reassessed as dyslexic at age 7, because he had been diagnosed before he had an opportunity to show the requisite discrepancy of two years between his chronological and reading age. In terms of literacy skills, by this stage, when prompted with the letter 's' at the beginning of a word such as 'says', he still failed to recognise the letter 's' at the end. His written performance was even worse, so that his teachers described him as the brightest boy in the class, but able to write less than the little Chinese boy who could not speak English. At this time, a placement in a special school was considered, but the local junior school decided they were prepared to take Matthew, despite his difficulties. It was an uphill struggle to ensure Matthew reached the appropriate reading level for his age, but we were fortunate enough to receive help from a friend, Tony Fryer, a junior school teacher with a belief in the merits of a structured approach. Tony taught Matthew on a voluntary basis for 2 hours each week, from his sixth birthday, until he reached secondary school, and in the process developed a lifelong interest in the anomaly of dyslexia. The work he set involved Matthew laboriously completing several exercises at home each week, always pitched at his level of understanding to maintain his interest in the task. As a young child, there were times when Matthew resented the level of commitment involved in this work, when other children his age were playing. The turning point came after about 6 months of instruction, when we took the gamble of allowing Matthew to decide for himself whether to continue with the lessons or not. Fortunately, he opted to continue. By the time he reached secondary school, his reading was adequate but slow, but he needed a further year in the special needs class to improve his writing and spelling skills.

Living in close proximity to the problem, I was inevitably faced with constant exposure to a whole series of dyslexic vagaries, such as confusion over times, days and even the general organisation of life. The pervasiveness of the deficit, in fact, again led me to question whether the problems we were dealing with could be dyslexic in origin. Most striking of all, in retrospect, was the clumsiness which led to a constant series of accidents ranging in severity from the regularly spilt drinks to a suspected broken back! But at the time, it was the simplest manifestations of dyslexia which appeared the most puzzling, in particular the problems with even the simplest rote learnt material. To illustrate this, at junior school, Matthew constantly muddled breakfast and supper, and he only grasped the difference when explicitly taught that breakfast was the first meal in the day, because it is then that you break your fast. At secondary school, he continued to exasperate his teachers with his forgetfulness, until they realised that this was just one manifestation of a more generalised memory problem. A memorable instance was the occasion when, having been sent home for a forgotten book, he simply forgot that he had put some sausages under the grill and set fire to the house.

Consequently, it soon became evident that, at least in Matthew's case, the dyslexic deficit was expressed in a whole range of areas more general than the traditionally accepted reading, spelling and language. At the same time, I was well aware that the most difficult part of coping with any handicap lies in accepting and coming to terms with a range of possible outcomes. Therefore, I set out to research the condition systematically, in as wide a range of dyslexic children of similar age as I could find. Eventually, I found myself armed with a battery of anecdotal evidence of generalised deficits in other dyslexic children – for instance, clumsiness and difficulty in rote learning – gleaned from my conversations with parents, teachers and children. It seemed that I was not alone in noting these bizarre manifestations of the problem, and clinicians in the field had a range of similar observations to report. On the other hand, it was clear that perceptions of dyslexia, unfortunately, remained very much dependent on the viewpoint of the observer. This is illustrated by a series of vignettes on the dyslexic child, drawn from interviews with parents and teachers and from school reports.

The teachers

Unsympathetic head (of dyslexic child, aged 7)
He's not dyslexic – he's just a silly little boy who won't concentrate for more than 10 seconds: what he needs is a good kick up the backside!

Exasperated (but supportive) teacher (of a 14 year old)
> This year Ben has put in the very minimum of effort. He arrives at lessons ill-prepared, his homework is rarely, if ever, handed in and his work is scrappily presented. He is his own worst enemy!

The parents

Baffled parent
> Alan just keeps losing things – he put his coat in the locker so it wouldn't get lost, but then he lost the key, and now he can't even remember which locker it was – he'd lose his own head if it wasn't joined on!

Depressed parent
> The depressing thing is that although we've gone over the word 20 times this weekend, he still doesn't seem to be any better at spelling it!

Desperate parent
> He's been in the remedial reading group for 5 years now, but I'm sure he's reading worse now than when he was 8 years old.

My need to understand the enigma of dyslexia led me to return to study as a mature student and altered the whole course of my life. An attempt to impose some meaning and order on such apparently disparate phenomena as these led me to the formulation of my research hypotheses. At the start of my PhD, I discussed these unexpected difficulties in rote learning with Rod Nicolson, who suggested that the underlying problem might be one of automatisation failure, and that this might best be tested experimentally using motor skills. This led us to challenge the dominant hypothesis that dyslexia is essentially a language-based problem, and consider instead that it might be a more generalised deficit in the acquisition of skills. The results of these analyses are presented in later chapters. Matthew, by the age of 14, would no longer be diagnosed as dyslexic in terms of his reading, but interestingly enough continued to show all the associated difficulties in spelling, clumsiness, memory and organisation that characterise the dyslexic. My personal involvement gave me the tenacity and temerity to follow through these hunches, which my thesis and subsequent research funding gave me a unique opportunity to explore in detail.

Our motivation in terms of dyslexia research has been to establish data for the range of types of skilled performance, which will provide a solid basis for researchers wishing to develop new theoretical approaches and for practitioners and parents interested in the wider manifestations of dyslexia. We are particularly fortunate to have contributions from Tim Miles, John Beech and John Rack, John Stein and Bill Lovegrove, and Regina Yap and Aryan van der Leij.

Preface

In this book we shall be discussing the symptoms and causes of 'specific developmental dyslexia', or dyslexia for short. Dyslexia is a term steeped in controversy, and even our apparently bland opening sentence conceals a multitude of disputes over terminology and definitions. One of the recurring themes of the wide-ranging research reported here is that dyslexia can take many forms, and we shall conclude that each of the current approaches to dyslexia research offers a further perspective on the underlying syndrome. There is a growing body of evidence that dyslexic children have problems not just in reading but in a range of skills, including several unrelated to reading. These findings are of considerable interest, in that they promise to provide a much more complete picture of the true problems of dyslexic children. In this book we have invited researchers from each of the major areas (language, phonology, vision, motor skill and learning) to present an overview of the dyslexia literature from their perspective. In this way we have derived a systematic, global view of the cognitive processes occurring in dyslexia, facilitating, we hope, objective discussion of the likely underlying cause or causes, and laying a foundation for consensual research progress. Consequently, in this preface we wish only to present an overview of some of the issues involved, and to preview the issues raised by the authors of each chapter. A fuller discussion will be presented in the final chapter.

DYSLEXIA

There is reasonable agreement about the general attributes of dyslexic children. They are 'children of average or above average intelligence who for no apparent reason read atrociously'. A more formal definition is 'a disorder in children who, despite conventional classroom experience, fail to attain the language skills of reading, writing and spelling commensurate with their intellectual abilities' (from the definition by the World Federation of Neurology, 1968). In other words, children of normal or above normal intelligence who, for some otherwise inexplicable reason, have inordinate problems learning to read and spell. One of the fascinating aspects of dyslexia research is that the syndrome manifests itself in many different ways, to the extent that, whatever a researcher's domain of interest, a dyslexic child will obligingly demonstrate interesting and unusual performance in that domain, thereby encouraging the researcher to believe that *the* explanation for the cause of dyslexia was nearly within his or her grasp! It has seemed at times to us that dyslexia is an equivalent of a Rorschach test – a complex jumble of symptoms whereof the interpretation indicates more about the researcher than the syndrome.

A brief historical review demonstrates both the range of possible explanations and the surprising swings in fashion which appear to characterise dyslexia research. Early writings on dyslexia were by James Hinshelwood (1917) a Glasgow eye surgeon, who used the term 'word blindness', and by the American neurologist Samuel Orton (1937), who advocated use of the term 'strephosymbolia' to indicate that the problem was not one of word blindness but of 'symbol twisting'. These early visually related discoveries set the pattern of research until the 1970s, when, following a seminal analysis by Frank Vellutino (1979), it was realised that the deficit was not just in visual processing, but also, and perhaps primarily, in processing of language. One of the major achievements of dyslexia researchers in the 1980s was to refine this concept of a linguistic deficit, developing the 'phonological deficit' theory which remains the consensus view of much of the dyslexia research community. Recently, new discoveries of abnormalities in the rapid processing of visual information, allied to findings of subtle difficulties in a wide range of skills, have cast doubt on the phonological deficit as the *only* cause of dyslexia.

As with any research area, it is often difficult to understand the reasoning underlying particular studies without understanding the general research background, and this is particularly the case in dyslexia research owing to the different perspectives and methods of different researchers. We felt therefore that it would be valuable to commission overview chapters from leading researchers in a number of areas with the intention of providing a broad yet detailed analysis of the 'state of the art' in dyslexia research. In order to give a feel for both established research findings and also the current research directions, we attempted to obtain two perspectives on each of three major areas of skill: language skill, visual skill and motor skill, together with a chapter which we contributed on learning and dyslexia; and an analysis of the requirements of taxonomic classification system for dyslexia. We believe that this collection of chapters provides one of the most comprehensive analyses ever produced of skill and its development in dyslexic children, and that it should prove a valuable reference for any practitioner wishing to know more about the signs of dyslexia or a researcher wishing to design a new study on dyslexia.

Despite the breadth of coverage, this book can only provide a partial view of dyslexia research and practice. An accessible and interesting general overview of dyslexia research and practice is provided by Tim and Elaine Miles, *Dyslexia: A hundred years on* (1990). A complete research review should include a series of chapters on the neurobiological and genetic underpinnings of dyslexia. There are interesting and important developments in these areas, but they are beyond the scope of this book. Several chapters provide brief references to this research, but the interested reader should consult a book devoted to these areas. Probably the most complete overview is provided by Drake Duane and Frank Gray, *The Reading Brain: The biological basis of dyslexia* (1989), in which five US research teams provide a complete overview of the major biological factors. In addition to research, of course, a complete treatise on dyslexia should include detailed analyses of diagnostic and remediation techniques. As will become clear from reading this book, the Duane and Gray book, or the book by Miles and Miles, diagnosis remains a thorny issue, with widespread dissatisfaction with current practice. By contrast, there appears to be reasonable consensus on support for dyslexic children, with the major requirements being 'do it well; do it early.' A valuable overview of a leading system is provided by Elaine Miles, *The Bangor Dyslexia Teaching System* (1989). A valuable review of computer-based teaching support is provided in Chris Singleton (ed.), *Computers and Literacy Skills* (1993). Finally, no analysis on dyslexia can be complete without a discussion of the political and legal aspects. A 'how to' manual for British parents is provided by Harry Chasty and John Friel, *Children with Special Needs: Assessment, law and practice: Caught in the act.* (London: Kingsley, 1991). Having provided a brief overview of what this book does not cover, we turn now to the positive aspects of coverage.

REFERENCES

Chasty, H. and Friel, J. (1991). *Children with Special Needs: Assessment, law and practice: Caught in the act.* London: Kingsley.

Duane, D.D. and Gray D.B. (Eds.), *The Reading Brain: The biological basis of dyslexia.* Parkton, MD: York Press.

Hinshelwood, J. (1917). *Congenital word blindness.* London: H.K. Lewis.

Just, M.A and Carpenter, P.A. (1987). *The Psychology of Reading and Language Comprehension.* Boston, MA: Allyn and Bacon.

Miles, T.R. and Miles, E. (1990). *Dyslexia: A hundred years on.* Milton Keynes: Open University Press.

Miles E. (1989) *The Bangor Dyslexia Teaching System.* London: Whurr.

Orton, S. T. (1937). *Reading, Writing and Speech Problems in Children.* New York: Norton.

Singleton, C. (Ed.), (1993).*Computers and Literacy Skills.* Hull: BDA Publications.

Vellutino, F.R. (1979). *Dyslexia: Theory and Research.* Cambridge, MA: MIT Press.

World Federation of Neurology (1968). *Report of Research Group on Dyslexia and World illiteracy.* Dallas: WFN.

OVERVIEW OF THE CHAPTERS

Part 1 Reading, phonological skills and dyslexia

Difficulties in learning to read are, of course, the litmus test for dyslexia, and it is therefore appropriate to begin this volume with two chapters which together provide a detailed overview of the skills involved in reading in both normal and dyslexic children.

One of the major achievements of international research on dyslexia in the 1980s was the emergence and refinement of the 'phonological deficit' hypothesis as a near-complete explanation of the problems dyslexic children face when learning to read. In brief, the hypothesis states that dyslexic children have an impairment in the ability to detect and process speech sounds (phonology), and that this impairment critically limits the skills which are a prerequisite for reading, such as the ability to detect rhymes, and, later, the ability to 'sound out' words and 'blend' sounds when trying to decipher the written word. John Rack has worked with groups in London, York and Colorado investigating the phonological deficit hypothesis, and has provided an authoritative overview of its current status. Rack's chapter is complemented by the chapter from John Beech, who provides a detailed review of current theoretical ideas on the processes of learning to read, ranging from studies of deaf children through connectionist models to an analysis of the difficulties dyslexic children experience with sublexical skills. The chapter ends by positing the hypothesis that children with dyslexia may have an intractable problem in acquiring phonological skill. The third chapter in this part, by Regina Yap and Aryan van der Leij, describes an empirical investigation of precisely this issue, directly examining the difficulties dyslexic children show in learning to read fluently. Of particular interest is their finding that, even when dyslexic children are matched with (younger) normal children of the same reading ability, the dyslexic children require more time to perceive a word when it is presented for a very brief period. Furthermore, a second, longitudinal study suggests that the ability to detect words under speeded conditions improves more slowly with time for the dyslexic children. The authors conclude that dyslexic children have greater than normal difficulties in automatising reading-related skills.

Part 2 Non-linguistic skills and their acquisition

The pioneers of dyslexia research, such as James Hinshelwood and Samuel Orton, believed that visual problems underlie the reading problems suffered by dyslexic children. Despite occasional demonstrations of visual anomalies, subsequent research has failed to substantiate this view, leading to a general belief that 'extensive evaluation suggests that visual deficits are unlikely to be the cause of most cases of dyslexia' (Just and Carpenter, 1987, p. 385). However, recent direct investigations of visual skill in Britain, Australia and the USA have led to striking findings of subtle visual deficits related to rapid processing of visual information, and of decreased binocular stability.

The first two chapters in this part provide overviews of the research in both these areas. Bill Lovegrove reviews the research on the deficits in transient visual processing (much of it undertaken in his laboratory in Wollongong, Australia), and John Stein presents evidence from his group in Oxford on instability of binocular control in dyslexic children, again interpreting the results in terms of problems in the transient visual system. The authors suggest that the deficits in visual skill may be part of a more general impairment in temporal aspects of sensory and motor performance.

One of the critical issues in dyslexia research is whether deficits in phonological skill and/or visual skill are sufficient to account for the range of deficits shown. The third chapter in this part, describing early work at our Sheffield laboratory, examines this issue directly. First, we summarise a series of studies in which we established that, although dyslexic children balanced as well as normal children of the same age under normal conditions, their balance deteriorated significantly when they were asked to undertake a simple task while balancing, whereas the normal children were unaffected. Furthermore, the dyslexic children balanced significantly worse than normal children when blindfolded. We interpret the results as indicating that the dyslexic children's balance skill is worse than that of normal children, but they are normally able to compensate for the skill deficit by 'conscious compensation'. These findings are of theoretical significance in that they reveal deficits in skill even when there is no overt phonological or visual component. A second set of studies investigated the process of skill acquisition, both for keyboard skills and for speed of reaction, establishing that dyslexic children show marked initial difficulties in skill, and that the difficulties persist even after many hours of practice.

Part 3 Issues in diagnosing dyslexia

In this final part we attempt to draw together the wide-ranging research described in Parts 1 and 2. Consequently, we felt it appropriate at this stage to provide a chapter from Tim Miles on the issues involved in diagnosing dyslexia, with particular reference to the question of how to cope with the problem that dyslexic children appear to be very heterogeneous, each showing a different constellation of difficulties. Professor Miles is, of course, particularly well placed to provide this overview, having extensive experience of diagnosis of dyslexia, and in particular having developed the Bangor Dyslexia Test, the first test to provide positive indicators of dyslexia rather than rely on discrepancy scores. He invokes the scientific concept of a 'taxonomy' as a major objective for dyslexia research, noting that if one were to have a 'strong' taxonomy for dyslexia, not only would diagnosis become easier and more objective, but also further progress would be made towards the objective of understanding the underlying causes. He criticises the traditional reliance on measures of reading and of IQ in defining dyslexia, and argues strongly for the use of positive measures rather than discrepancy scores. He concludes the chapter by outlining the requirements for an adequate taxonomy, arguing that phonological deficits in the presence of good reasoning skills remain the major indicator, but that deficits in speed of processing may well be a useful supplementary indicator.

The final chapter provides a summary of recently completed research in our laboratory which addresses directly the issues raised by Miles in terms of heterogeneity and diagnosis of dyslexia, together with issues implicit in many of the other chapters. We administered a series of tasks, designed to tap the range of 'primitive' skills (phonological skill, memory, speed of processing, motor skill and balance), to groups of dyslexic and matched control children. This was intended to investigate the issue of whether there really were deficits in all these skills, and if so, which were the most severe. Interestingly, deficits were obtained across the range of skills tested, with balance and phonological skill deficits being among the most severe. Comparison with a group of non-dyslexic 'slow learner' children suggested that they were even more severely impaired on phonological skill, but less impaired on balance. The results suggest promising lines of enquiry for further developments in theoretical understanding and in diagnostic methods.

GUIDE FOR READERS

Each of the chapters can be read as a self-contained overview of the literature or a set of empirical studies. It should be noted that we have deliberately set out to obtain contributions from eminent researchers representing the range of major theoretical research themes in dyslexia. As editors, we have been able to have the last word in the book by means of the final chapter, but this should not be taken to imply that most dyslexia researchers, or even the contributors to this volume, would agree with the conclusions we reach. One of the fascinations of dyslexia research is that much progress is currently being made, and theoretical positions are in a state of flux. Our intention in this volume is to collate and present the information currently available on dyslexia and skill. It is the reader's prerogative to select whichever theoretical approach appears most congenial.

Contributors

Dr John Beech, University of Leicester

John. R. Beech, PhD, is a lecturer in psychology at the University of Leicester. He is a fellow of the British Psychological Society, Treasurer of the BPS Cognitive Section, and series editor of the NFER-Nelson assessment library. His area of research is the development of reading skills and he has been a university lecturer for 18 years.

Dr Angela Fawcett, University of Sheffield

Following experience of dyslexia in her family and active participation in the British Dyslexia Association, Angela Fawcett was a mature entrant to academia, and has a BA and PhD in Psychology from the University of Sheffield. Her research on dyslexia, in collaboration with Rod Nicolson, started from the premiss that dyslexic children have broad deficits in skill learning and automatisation, and provides a different perspective from those normally adopted.

Professor Aryan van der Leij, Free University of Amsterdam

Aryan van der Leij has a degree in Educational Psychology and a PhD in the area of special reading disabilities from the Free

University of Amsterdam, where he has been Professor of Special Education since 1986. He has published extensively in Dutch and English on reading and reading difficulties, and, in conjunction with his colleagues, has developed the COTAL suite of computer-based reading tests.

Professor William Lovegrove, University of Wollongong

Bill Lovegrove is Chair of the Department of Psychology and Dean of the Graduate Faculty at the University of Wollongong, Australia. He has been researching possible visual processing deficits in dyslexia for over twelve years. His research suggests that many dyslexics do have a specific visual deficit. His current research interests concern how this visual deficit relates to other deficits experienced by dyslexics and their possible remedial implications.

Professor T. R. Miles, University of Wales, Bangor

Tim Miles is Emeritus Professor of Psychology, University of Wales Bangor and a Vice-President of the British Dyslexia Association. He has published academic books on dyslexia and books for parents and teachers, and is author of the Bangor Dyslexia Test for assessment of dyslexia. He has unique experience with dyslexia at all ages, including university students, who are attracted to Bangor by the Dyslexia Unit and the support available therein.

Dr Rod Nicolson, University of Sheffield

Having gained a first degree in mathematics and a PhD in Psychology from Cambridge University, Rod Nicolson is now senior lecturer in Cognitive Psychology at the University of Sheffield. He has had a lifetime interest in human learning, and has published articles and books in areas ranging from mathematical psychology through intelligent tutoring systems to university teaching methods. His research in dyslexia, in collaboration with Angela Fawcett, adopts a learning perspective.

Dr John Rack, University of York

John Rack has experience of dyslexia in both children and adults, using traditional and computer-based methodology, and in his work on the Colorado family study, he was involved in both the genetic and the remedial aspects of dyslexia. His chapter was completed whilst working at the University of York on a research project investigating phonological awareness in a longitudinal study of the development of 4–5 year olds. Recently, he has been appointed to the Dyslexia Institute (Staines, England).

Dr John Stein, University of Oxford

John Stein trained as a neurologist at Oxford, Leicester and St Thomas' Hospital, London, before becoming lecturer in Neurophysiology, Oxford University, and fellow and tutor in Medicine, Magdalen College, Oxford. His interest has therefore had a clinical perspective. He is interested in the visual guidance of movement, which he investigates by means of computer simulations, recording and inactivation experiments in monkeys trained to perform visuomanual tracking tasks, and the analysis of visuomotor disorders in neurological patients and dyslexic children.

Dr Regina Yap, Free University of Amsterdam

Regina Yap has recently completed her doctoral research in Psychology at the Free University of Amsterdam, supervised by Aryan van der Leij, in which she undertook an extensive series of studies of the speed and automaticity of reading skills in dyslexic and normal children. In addition to her work on dyslexia and education, she has strong interest in hypermedia.

PART 1

Phonological skills, reading and dyslexia

Difficulties in learning to read are, of course, the litmus test for dyslexia, and it is therefore appropriate to begin this volume with two chapters which together provide a detailed overview of the skills involved in reading in normal and dyslexic children. One of the major achievements of international research on dyslexia in the 1980s was the emergence and refinement of the 'phonological deficit' hypothesis as a near-complete explanation of the problems dyslexic children face when learning to read. In brief, the hypothesis states that dyslexic children have an impairment in the ability to detect and process speech sounds (phonology), and that this impairment critically limits the skills which are a prerequisite for reading, such as the ability to detect rhymes, and, later, the ability to 'sound out' words and 'blend' sounds when trying to decipher the written word.

John Rack has worked with groups in London, York and Colorado investigating the phonological deficit hypothesis, and has provided an authoritative overview of its current status. Rack makes it his task to assess the adequacy of the phonological deficit hypothesis in terms of the four criteria of *specificity* (why is the problem specific to reading-related skills rather than more general cognitive abilities?), *causality* (are phonological deficits the cause, a consequence or a correlate of the reading problems?), *process* (can one specify the process by which phonological deficits result in reading problems) and *variation* (are differences in severity of phonological deficit sufficient to account for individual variations in reading difficulty?). Considering first the issue of specificity, Rack presents a range of studies of phonological deficits, including short-term memory, verbal repetition, long-term memory and naming, thereby explaining and establishing the case for the phonological deficit hypothesis. In an investigation of causality, he then goes on to consider more direct assessments of phonological skills, including rhyming and phonological awareness, and their role in learning to read. Next he links these deficits to evidence from the specific difficulties identified in dyslexics, emphasising nonword reading deficits and error analysis. In an important theoretical analysis of the processes involved, Rack links these findings to a model of reading development, considering in particular the role of phonetic cues in early reading. He argues that dyslexic children are able to make use of limited phonetic cues in reading, but that they would have continuing difficulties with the more complex processes of grapheme–phoneme mapping. Rack concludes that the phonological deficit hypothesis fulfils the criteria for a difficulty in processing outside the realm of reading, which impacts upon the development of literacy skills.

In the second chapter, John Beech focuses on Rack's third issue, the processes by which dyslexic children acquire reading abnormally, and presents a thorough and detailed overview of current theories and data on children learning to read, considering the development of reading skills in normal readers. He draws on 'dual-route' theories of reading, which assume that a word may be read either as a whole via visual features (the lexical or logographic route) or assembled from the series of word segments such as the individual graphemes (the sublexical route). The logographic route is typically found in the early stages of reading, whereas the sublexical route is dependent on word segmentation and blending using phonological cues. A major issue considered is whether or not dyslexic children who rely predominantly on logographic (whole word) reading are able to become fluent readers without acquiring sublexical skills. First, he considers the evidence for the development of reading in a population of deaf children, who are limited to the logographic skills in their route to reading. He goes on to discuss connectionist simulations of reading; case studies of acquired dyslexia in mature readers with minimal sublexical skill; and the development of automaticity in normal children. Then he considers the evidence for the development of fluency in dyslexia, first in adults, and then in a longitudinal case-study of reading with minimal sublexical involvement.

Beech next discusses the development of sublexical skills (that is, skills in processing the components of words), in particular the development of reading and phonology in normally achieving readers, and presents a meta-analysis of the effects of training on segmentation and blending. He considers the unit of analysis in the sublexical route, whether simply grapheme to phoneme or onset and rime. Beech explores the issue of resistance to developing lexical skills in a small subgroup of dyslexics, who are unable or unwilling to use this route. He discusses the lack of interaction between lexical and sublexical processes in training studies, suggesting that these might represent either the impact of cumulative deficits, or an intractable resistance to training in sublexical skills. He concludes that a subset of dyslexic children may be limited to reading by analogy, missing out the sublexical route, and outlines a remediation strategy which could be used.

The third chapter in this part, by Regina Yap and Aryan Van der Leij, examines an issue highlighted by both Rack and Beech, namely the question of whether, given extensive training, dyslexic children are able to acquire normal fluency of reading, or whether there is indeed some intractable problem within the processes involved. Rather than phonological skill, however, they focus directly on the time taken to perceive a written word. Of particular interest is their finding that, even when dyslexic Dutch children were matched with (younger) normal children on reading ability, the dyslexic children required more time to perceive a word when the words were presented for very brief periods. Furthermore, a second, longitudinal study suggested that this ability to detect words under speeded conditions improved more slowly with time for the dyslexic children. The authors conclude that dyslexic children have greater than normal difficulties in acquiring fluency in reading-related skills, a conclusion consonant with the positions taken by Rack and by Beech. Their account, in terms of difficulties of automatisation of skill, is somewhat different from that provided by the phonological deficit hypothesis, and provides a valuable link to the material reviewed in Part 2 of this volume.

CHAPTER 1

Dyslexia: The Phonological Deficit Hypothesis

John P. Rack

INTRODUCTION

The present chapter is concerned with the relationship between phonological skills and specific reading difficulties or dyslexia. In particular, it is concerned with the hypothesis that a deficit in the processing of phonological information – information about the sounds of words – is at the root of most dyslexics' reading and spelling problems. This is the theory that is here called the Phonological Deficit Hypothesis. Many variants of the theory exist (e.g., Bradley and Bryant, 1983; 1985; Brady, 1986; Frith, 1981; 1985; Goswami and Bryant, 1990; Liberman and Shankweiler, 1979; Mann, 1984; Olson *et al.*, 1990; Shankweiler *et al.*, 1979; Snowling, 1987; Stanovich, 1988; Vellutino and Scanlon, 1987), some of which are more concerned with normal development and some more with reading difficulties. Before reviewing some of the recent evidence that supports the phonological deficit hypothesis, it is useful to discuss the general problems for all deficit accounts of dyslexia and to show how these have been addressed, with some success, in the literature on phonological skills. As we shall see later,

some people have argued that it is now the right time to redefine
dyslexia to reflect the central role of phonological processes in its
aetiology (Catts, 1989; Siegel, 1988). A major theme of the present
chapter is to identify the type of evidence which would be necessary
for such a redefinition and to see how well the evidence supporting
phonological deficit theory goes towards meeting these
requirements.

Dyslexia has typically been defined, negatively, by applying a set
of exclusionary criteria. Thus a dyslexic person must have average
or above average intelligence; adequate opportunities to learn to
read; no sensory or neurological damage and no psychiatric or
emotional problems (Critchley, 1970; Stanovich, 1986; Vellutino,
1979). Dyslexic children are therefore something of a puzzle: they
are poor readers and spellers, but there is no obvious reason why this
should be so. Indeed, the lack of any obvious explanation leads
some to deny the existence of the condition itself.

Most people, however, now accept that dyslexia is a specific and
sometimes subtle difficulty with aspects of learning or information
processing. The highly specific processing difficulties shown by
dyslexic children are of great interest to psychologists who wish to
understand the components (or modules) of cognitive abilities. The
existence of specific deficits, along with evidence for specific
abilities, is powerful evidence for a 'componential' theory of
intellectual functioning (see Sternberg, 1982, for further discussion).
It would be very informative if it could be shown that there is a
particular cognitive deficit which affects reading and spelling skills
but has a relatively minor influence on other intellectual abilities. In
this spirit, a large amount of research has been directed at
identifying the specific cognitive deficits that 'go along' with
dyslexia, and which may be at the root of the problem.

Understanding the *unexpected* or unusual problems that cause
dyslexia is an important goal for practical as well as theoretical
purposes. It has considerable significance for dyslexic people
themselves and for their parents and teachers who may feel
responsible for their children's difficulties. An understanding of the
underlying cause of dyslexia is also an important first stage in
devising appropriate remedial programmes. Remedial programmes
need both to target the areas of weakness and to seek ways around
severe difficulties which may be resistant to teaching.

An understanding of the causes of dyslexia should lead to a

more satisfactory (positive) definition of dyslexia. Such a definition would allow identification of people who have behavioural or emotional problems at school *because* they have specific reading and spelling problems. Their behaviour may be the result of the unsympathetic treatment that they have received from parents or teachers, or it may be their way of avoiding confronting their reading and spelling problems. Either way, such people would not meet the exclusionary criteria for dyslexia although they may have reading and spelling difficulties for the same reasons as dyslexics. Rather than relying on the exclusionary criteria, it would therefore be preferable to identify dyslexia using a set of *positive symptoms* (Catts, 1989; Fletcher and Morris, 1986; Miles, 1983).

A final, important practical consequence of a proper understanding of the causes of dyslexia is that it should facilitate early detection of potential difficulties. If we know which cognitive difficulties are at the root of dyslexia, it may be possible to screen for those difficulties at an early stage and possibly prevent reading and spelling problems from arising.

Thus, deficit accounts of dyslexia are very attractive since the theoretical and practical consequences are extensive. Early research focused on the role of visual-processing difficulties, but a comprehensive review by Vellutino (1979) showed that much of the evidence could be interpreted in terms of verbal difficulties. Attention then shifted to verbal, and specifically phonological, skills and this is the area receiving the greatest research attention today. Interest in visual and other skills remains, as the other chapters of this book testify, and, as will become apparent, the present hypothesis does not deny the importance of some of these factors. Before going on to consider the evidence relating to the phonological deficit theory, we turn to the general problems for all deficit accounts of dyslexia. These we may term specificity, causality, process, and variation.

The nature of the current exclusionary definition of dyslexia dictates that the relevant underlying deficit must be highly *specific*. A general explanation, in terms of gross differences in visual or phonological differences, or in terms of general rule acquisition skill (Morrison and Manis, 1983), is hard to reconcile with the definition of dyslexia as a *specific* learning difficulty. Such global deficits would be expected to influence abilities more generally and therefore lead to learning problems across a wide range of cognitive

Dyslexia in Children

domains. (See Stanovich, 1986, for an elaboration of this argument.) A slightly different possibility is that an underlying deficit is very mild. It may therefore go undetected except in particularly demanding circumstances. In either case, deficit accounts need to explain why some tasks (notably reading and spelling) pose more problems for dyslexic individuals than are posed by other tasks.

The second challenge for deficit accounts is to determine whether poor reading is a *cause* or a *consequence* of the associated deficit. Learning to read gives children a source of knowledge and a set of procedures (or strategies) that they may use in tasks that are not obviously concerned with reading. An example of this is judgements about the number of sounds in words, which is strongly influenced by knowledge of how the words are spelled (Ehri and Wilce, 1980). Thus it is not unreasonable to suppose that good and poor readers (or dyslexics) may differ on some tasks because the better readers have more skills and knowledge available to them.

A further problem is that associated deficits may not be directly related to the reading problem in dyslexia but both may be manifestations of a third, more fundamental, deficit. In this case, particular difficulties may tend to co-occur with dyslexia but it would be wrong to argue that they are the cause (or indeed the consequence) of dyslexia. Their co-occurrence may be useful diagnostically, but it may not help to understand the nature of dyslexia or the appropriate remedial action.

The problems of determining the direction of causation between two associated variables emphasises the need to understand the nature of such relationships in terms of *processes* or mechanisms. We need to know how a particular skill comes to influence another skill, or how a skill deficiency leads to a further skill deficiency – in this case, dyslexia. To develop such an understanding is clearly a difficult task. It demands the integration of information from a wide range of studies and theories. The most progress towards such a process-oriented deficit account has been made by those studying the role of phonological skills in reading (see Hulme and Snowling, 1991). A summary of this progress will be provided here, along with a review of some of the relevant evidence.

The final problem for all deficit accounts is that of individual *variation*. Many people have argued that dyslexia is a heterogeneous category and that distinct subtypes of dyslexics exist (e.g., Boder, 1973; Seymour, 1986). An obvious possibility, therefore, is that the different subtypes are caused by different underlying deficits. However, other people have questioned whether dyslexics do fit more easily into two (or more) categories rather than one (Olson *et al.*, 1985; Rack, Snowling and Olson, 1992; Treiman and Hirsh-Pasek, 1985). Individual differences clearly exist in reading and spelling behaviour, however, it has yet to be shown that these differences relate to skills outside the reading system, except, that is, to phonological skills. A possibility that has been raised by Rack, Snowling and Olson (1992; see also, Snowling, 1987) is that an underlying phonological deficit may be the root cause of nearly all dyslexics' difficulties, but that the other skills available to them influence the degree to which they are able to develop reading skills despite their phonological difficulties.

In order to meet the above-mentioned challenges for deficit accounts of dyslexia, we have to draw on information from different types of study using different methodologies. Here we shall discuss data that show that dyslexics have phonological deficits outside the domain of reading, we shall discuss data concerned with the reading processes used by dyslexics, and we shall discuss data on the normal development of reading together with current theoretical conceptualisations of reading development.

DYSLEXICS' DEFICITS IN PHONOLOGICAL SKILLS

Short-term memory deficits

One of the most reliable and often-quoted associated characteristics of developmental dyslexia is an inefficiency in short-term memory. For example, Digit Span scores on the Wechsler Intelligence Scales for Children (WISC) tend to be lower for poor readers – even when compared to normal readers matched on overall intelligence (Rugel, 1974). Confirmation that phonological processes are used in such short-term memory tasks has been obtained by comparing performance on rhyming letters (e.g., B C G P and T) with non-rhyming letters (e.g., H K S L and Q). The finding that performance is worse on the phonologically confusable letters (Baddeley, 1966;

Conrad, 1964) suggests that information is held in short-term memory in a phonological form (many people also have a subjective experience of using 'inner speech' in such tasks). Early reports suggested that dyslexics may not use phonological codes in short-term memory to the same extent as normal readers, since they tended not to show such a large difference between rhyming and non-rhyming letters (Shankweiler *et al.*, 1979; Siegel and Linder, 1984; Siegel and Ryan, 1988). However, it was subsequently shown that dyslexics show the same 'phonetic confusability effect' when they are compared with younger normal readers matched on memory span (Hall *et al.*, 1983; Johnston, Rugg and Scott, 1987) or reading level (Holligan and Johnston, 1988). These findings confirm that dyslexics do make use of phonological codes in short-term memory, but they are less efficient in doing so and hence have more limited short-term memory capacities.

Studies of good and poor readers – especially when the groups are matched on reading level – confirm that there is an association between short-term memory and reading ability and they are strongly suggestive of a role for short-term memory deficits in dyslexic children's difficulties. However, this association does not tell us very much about the direction of any causal relationship that might exist, or, indeed, whether the association is mediated by a third common causal factor. To help answer these questions we must turn to longitudinal studies of children across the whole range of abilities.

Jorm *et al.* (1984) tested the memory abilities of 5-year-old children just starting school. Their memory scores were found to be predictive of later success in reading, even after controlling for general factors such as IQ and age on entry to school. A similar finding was reported by Mann and Liberman (1984). These studies are therefore highly suggestive of a causal link between memory span and success in learning to read. However, a more recent study by Ellis (1991) has shown that reading ability scores are predictive of later short-term memory scores. One possible reason why this might be so is that reading experience gives children an additional source of knowledge about words (spelling knowledge) which they can use as the basis for a memory code (Frick, 1984; Rack, 1985). Another possibility is that both measures are influenced by a third common factor and that this factor has varying relationships with memory and reading at different points in time. One candidate for such a third variable which we shall discuss later is phonological processing skill.

Bryant and Goswami (1987) have argued that training studies are necessary in order to disentangle complex relationships between variables such as memory and reading. A training study would have to alter the short-term memory abilities of one group of children and demonstrate the consequence of this manipulation on later reading. In practice it would be very hard to train short-term memory in isolation although, as we shall see, some training programmes may inadvertently influence memory abilities along with other skills.

Verbal repetition

It should be simpler to repeat a single word than to repeat a sequence of words in the correct order. Yet dyslexics are reported to have such difficulties especially on long polysyllabic words (Miles, 1983) and on pseudowords or 'nonsense words'. For example, Snowling (1981) found that dyslexics were worse than normal reading level-matched readers at repeating pseudowords such as *bagmivishent*. In a subsequent study, Snowling *et al.* (1986) replicated the finding of a nonword repetition deficit and also included a noise manipulation (stimuli were heard in differing levels of background noise) in order to see whether the dyslexics were differentially affected. If so, this would suggest that their difficulty lay at the perceptual level. Both groups were equally affected by noise, so Snowling *et al.* concluded that the problem lay with the processes of speech-segmentation.

A slightly different view of nonsense word repetition ability was taken by Gathercole and Baddeley (1989). They conducted a longitudinal study to assess the influence of nonword repetition ability on the acquisition of spoken vocabulary, as measured by the British Picture Vocabulary Test. The children's nonword repetition ability at age 5 predicted oral vocabulary one year later; it was actually a better predictor of oral vocabulary at age 6 than was oral vocabulary at age 5. Gathercole and Baddeley (1989) take the view that the nonword repetition task is primarily a measure of short-term memory and this is why it has a role in vocabulary acquisition. However, there are other interpretations of this finding (see Hulme and Snowling, 1991). One possibility is that nonsense word repetition skill has its influence on oral vocabulary via reading ability. As Snowling's studies suggest, nonsense word reading is related to reading ability so it would be possible that the children with good nonword repetition skill became the better readers and therefore developed larger oral vocabularies. Although Gathercole and Baddeley's results are ambiguous they are important because they demonstrate that phonological skills directly or indirectly shape the development of oral vocabulary.

Long-term memory

A number of studies have compared dyslexic and normal readers on measures of long-term memory. Many models of memory predict that short-term memory difficulties would impact upon the encoding of information in long-term memory. Therefore we may expect to find that dyslexics have long-term memory difficulties as a consequence of their short-term memory limitations. A study by Bauer and Emhert (1984) demonstrated this pattern of difficulties. In a list-learning test the items presented in the middle of the list are remembered least well; the final items are usually remembered better because they are still in short-term memory (recency effect) and the first items are usually remembered better because they have had more time to be transferred into long-term memory (primacy effect). Transfer into long-term memory is partly related to efficiency in rehearsing information during presentation of later items (see Baddeley, 1986; Rack and Snowling, 1985, for further explanation). Bauer and Emhert (1984) found that dyslexics showed a reduced primacy effect indicating that they are less efficient in transferring information into long-term memory.

Dyslexics' memory performance can be improved by encouraging rehearsal (Cohen and Netley, 1981). However, there is evidence from other studies that some difficulties cannot be attributed to failure to rehearse. For example, Byrne and Shea (1979) showed that dyslexics made more false positive responses (i.e., saying an item had been presented when it had not) to semantically similar items in a continuous monitoring task. In contrast, normal readers made more false positives to phonologically similar items. This finding suggests that dyslexics may attend to different properties of stimuli and/or encode stimuli in a different manner in long-term memory. Rack (1985) directly tested this possibility using a cued-recall experiment. In Rack's (1985) study, subjects saw or heard pairs of words about which they had to make rhyme judgements. They were given one of the words from each pair (the cue) later and asked to recall the other member of the pair (the target). Normal readers and dyslexics showed an effect of phonological similarity, recalling targets from the rhyming pairs better than those from the non-rhyming pairs. However, the dyslexics showed this effect to a reduced extent, especially when the pairs were presented visually. This finding provides support for the idea that dyslexics do not always make use of a phonological code for storing information in memory. Rack argued that it should be possible to demonstrate that the dyslexics made use of different codes to a greater extent than the younger normals who were matched on reading age. Evidence that they did was obtained by comparing performance on the cues which were visually (orthographically) similar to their intended targets (*head–dead*) with those cue–target pairs that were visually different (*rope–soap*). Again, both groups made use of the visual similarity of the words and were better able to recall the visually similar pairs than the visually different pairs. However, this time the dyslexics showed the effect to a greater extent, suggesting that they were making more use of a visual memory code than the normal readers.

In summary, the studies by Rack (1985) and Byrne and Shea (1979) along with others (e.g., Holligan and Johnston, 1988; Mark *et al.*, 1977; Olson *et al.*, 1984), provide clear evidence that dyslexics make less use of phonological coding in long-term memory.

Naming

One possible explanation for dyslexics' phonological memory difficulties is that the phonological information stored in memory is difficult to retrieve or is poorly coded. These difficulties would lead to difficulties 'finding the right word' and to mispronunciations of some words. Such mispronunciations are indeed a characteristic of many dyslexic children (Miles, 1983). Word-finding difficulties can be detected by asking children to name pictures of familiar, but perhaps infrequently encountered, objects such as a xylophone or stethoscope. Katz (1986) found dyslexics to be worse than normal readers of the same age when naming simple pictures, especially those with long and infrequently encountered names. Interpretation of this study is complicated by the fact that the dyslexics and normal comparison group differed in terms of reading ability. It is not therefore possible to exclude the possibility that the naming differences were caused by differing reading level. Such an influence is quite possible since it is by reading books that children are likely to encounter unusual words and become practised in retrieving their spoken forms from long-term memory.

A study by Snowling, van Wagtendonk and Stafford (1988) included a reading level-matched control to avoid this difficulty. The dyslexics were found to perform at a similar level to the younger children. This finding provides further evidence of naming difficulties in dyslexia but it does not clarify question of the relationship between reading and naming. In a second experiment Snowling *et al.* compared dyslexics and normal readers who were similar in age and who were matched on a measure of vocabulary knowledge. In this way, they could be sure that any differences that arose would not be due simply to differing vocabulary knowledge that may have been a consequence of differences in reading level and experience. Despite their similar vocabulary knowledge (confirmed with a second measure) the dyslexics were found to make more errors in naming pictures. This result shows that dyslexics have a quite specific deficit in word-naming relative to their knowledge of word-meanings. However, there is no clear evidence to show whether these naming difficulties precede the reading difficulties or, indeed, whether the two types of problem have a third, common cause.

Phonological skills

The evidence that has been considered up to now is consistent with the view that dyslexics have a fundamental phonological processing deficit which impacts upon their skills in a variety of verbal tasks. Poor performances in short-term memory, long-term memory, picture naming and verbal repetition would all be consistent with a deficiency in the use of phonologically-based information. We shall next consider some of the studies that have tried to assess phonological skills more directly in order to evaluate their role in reading development and reading difficulty.

Rhyme

Before they learn to read, many children engage in rhyming and word-sound games that depend on sensitivity to the sound-structure of words. In a series of studies, Bradley and Bryant (1978; 1983; 1985) investigated the hypothesis that sensitivity to rhyme and alliteration might play a causal role in the development of reading abilities and disabilities. Bradley and Bryant (1978) compared dyslexic and reading level-matched normal readers on a series of tasks in which children had to indicate which was the odd one out in a sequence of words such as *sun sock see rag* or *cap map bag rap*. Dyslexic readers were worse than reading-level matched normal readers on these tasks, which suggests that their lack of sensitivity to rhyme and alliteration may have had a role in their reading difficulties. Consistent evidence was obtained by Rack (1985), who found that dyslexic readers were at the same level as younger reading level-matched controls on a simple rhyme-judgement task. Using a similar procedure, Holligan and Johnston (1988) found that dyslexics were worse at making rhyme judgements. These studies therefore establish that dyslexics have difficulties with the apparently simple task of deciding whether two words rhyme or detecting the non-rhyming word in a short list.

In an extension of their initial study Bradley and Bryant (1983; 1985) set out to determine whether sensitivity to rhyme and alliteration had a causal role in reading development. A sample of 403 4–5-year-olds were given the Bradley and Bryant (1978) sound-categorisation task and their progress in reading and spelling was monitored over a period of four years. Subjects who had begun to learn to read at the start of the project were excluded so that Bradley and Bryant could be sure that the sound-categorisation scores were not confounded with reading ability. After accounting for general factors such as IQ, age at initial testing and memory for the word lists, sound-categorisation accounted for 4–10% of the variance in reading and 6–10% of the variance in spelling. The influence of sound-categorisation skill appeared to be fairly specific since it accounted for less of the variance in later mathematics ability.

The second part of Bradley and Bryant's longitudinal study involved an intervention programme which was given to a sample of 65 children who had poor sound-categorisation skills. The children were divided into four groups each of which was given a different type of training: (1) sound-categorisation training; (2) sound-categorisation training supported by concrete materials (plastic letters); (3) semantic categorisation training; (4) a no-treatment control. After two years, the effects of training were evaluated by standardised tests of reading and spelling. Sound-categorisation training seemed to have a beneficial effect on later reading and spelling, but it was only significantly better than the semantic categorisation control when plastic letters were also used as part of the training.

Bradley and Bryant's results are impressive in their demonstration of a causal link between sound-categorisation ability and reading. Two reservations need to be noted, however. The first is that sound-categorisation training was not successful unless it was integrated with letter knowledge. This may lead some to argue that the children in this condition were, effectively, being taught to read and their greater progress is therefore unsurprising. (Recall that the logic of deficit accounts of dyslexia is that a skill unrelated to reading is the origin of the difficulties.) Second, it is not entirely clear what the sound-categorisation task is measuring. Wagner and Torgeson (1987) suggest that it may be a better test of memory than of phonological skills. Others have noted that the predictive success of the Bradley and Bryant task may depend on its complexity (Rack, Hulme and Snowling, 1993).

Phonological awareness

A multitude of tasks has been used to measure what is often called *phonemic* awareness. Phonemic awareness refers to the awareness of words as sequences of discrete phonemes such as /c/ /a/ /t/. Tasks to measure phonemic awareness include counting phonemes, deleting phonemes, substituting phonemes and dividing words into phonemes. Other tasks are concerned with awareness of larger units of sounds within words; these include counting syllables in words, deleting syllables and dividing words into various subsyllabic units. Rhyming ability could also be included in this latter category of skills. There continues to be controversy about the number of factors that are needed to account for children's abilities on these various tasks (Goswami and Bryant, 1990; Lundberg Frost and Peterson, 1988; Stanovich *et al.*, 1984; Yopp, 1988) which cannot be resolved at this time.

Many of the phonemic awareness tasks have been used primarily in studies of normal reading development. Much of the impetus for these studies came from workers at the Haskins Laboratories who were among the first to stress the role of language processes in learning to read and to show that poor readers had difficulties on these tasks (for reviews see Gleitman and Rozin, 1977; Liberman and Shankweiler, 1979; Liberman *et al.*, 1974; Rozin and Gleitman, 1977; Shankweiler and Liberman, 1990). These studies were important in demonstrating a close association between reading ability and phonemic awareness tasks, but they could not reveal much about the nature of this association. As we have seen already, the influence could be in either direction or mediated by a third common variable. Longitudinal and reading level-matched studies are therefore needed to help explain the relationship.

One of the few studies to compare dyslexics and reading level-matched normal readers on a test of phonemic awareness was reported by Olson *et al.* (1989). The task used by Olson *et al.* was a 'Pig Latin' game in which the initial phoneme of a word had to be moved to the end of the word and the sound 'ay' added (pig therefore becomes ig-pay). Dyslexic readers were worse than reading level-matched normal readers on this task. In similar vein, Olson, Rack and Forsberg (1990) have reported that dyslexics are worse than reading level-matched normal readers on a phoneme-deletion task in which subjects have to remove a phoneme from a nonword to produce a real word (e.g., glamp without the /g/). These reading level-matched studies are important because they show that performance on 'phoneme awareness' tasks is not simply a function of reading level. The studies are consistent with the view that dyslexics are able to acquire reading skills despite poor phonological awareness skills, but that phonological awareness difficulties make reading acquisition more difficult for them (see Rack, Snowling and Olson, 1992, for an elaboration of this view).

Longitudinal studies of the role of phonological awareness have been fraught with methodological problems (see Rack, Hulme and Snowling, 1993; Wagner and Torgeson, 1987). For example, a study by Stanovich, Cunningham and Cramer (1984) demonstrated that performance on a range of phonemic awareness tasks was highly predictive of later reading ability. The phonological measures were better predictors than general IQ which is often held to be one of the best predictors of academic success. However, the children in this study had already begun to learn to read at the time when their phonological skills were measured. It is therefore possible that the children with better phonological skills were *already* the better readers at the first time of testing. We cannot therefore conclude that good phonological awareness caused good reading. A similar problem applies to the studies of Lundberg, Olofson and Wall (1980); Mann (1984) and Mann and Liberman (1984).

Better evidence for the importance of phonological skills in reading acquisition comes from a training study reported by Lundberg, Frost and Peterson (1988). 235 Danish kindergarten children were given phonological awareness training and 155 children served as controls. All the subjects were given a battery of linguistic and metalinguistic tests at the beginning and at the end of their kindergarten year. In the intervening period the experimental group received daily 15–20-minute training sessions designed to promote phonological awareness. The control group were given no special attention but followed the normal pre-school activity programme. Neither group was given any direct training in reading. Using this design, it was possible to assess the effects of 'pure' phonological awareness training. In most other cases, phonological awareness training occurs alongside reading development and the outcome may well be a function of the interaction of these activities.

Lundberg *et al.* needed to first establish that they could alter children's phonological abilities without the support of written materials. The training programme consisted of a carefully constructed series of games and exercises. This began with simple listening games and rhyming games; moving through segmentation of sentences into words, words into syllables; and on to segmentation of initial phonemes and finally phonemes within words. The experimental group did indeed outscore the control group on the post-test measures of phonological abilities despite the fact that the control group had slightly (but significantly) higher scores on the pre-test. In contrast, general language comprehension and letter knowledge increased equally for both groups over the training period. The effects of phonological skills training were thus highly specific to the phonological domain. This is important since the experimental group might have showed greater improvements across the range of tests simply because they received special attention and the control group did not. Phonological skill was also assessed three months into the first year in school using a different set of tasks. Differences favouring the experimental group remained, indicating that the effects of training were persistent.

The effect of training was observed on a composite measure of seven phonological tests. Confirmatory factor analysis showed that a 2-factor structure provided a good fit to the data. One factor consisted of the three tasks requiring a phonemic segmentation and another consisted of the three measures requiring word and syllable segmentation. The two factors were moderately correlated at 0.40. Training had the greatest effects on the phoneme-segmentation tasks, whereas the effects on syllable-level tasks and the rhyming task were modest in comparison. The lack of a strong effect for rhyming may be due to the fact that both groups were already fairly good at rhyming before the intervention began.

The more permanent effects of the phonemic awareness training were investigated by measuring reading and spelling some 7 months into the children's first year in school and again in the middle of their second year. The experimental group outscored the control group on reading and spelling at both follow-up times although the differences in reading in grade 1 were not significant. In contrast, the control group outscored the experimental group on a test of mathematics that had been given in the first year. This important control test indicates that the training had not had a global effect on all school subjects but it had specifically affected the targeted skills of reading and spelling.

Lundberg *et al.*'s study is important because it demonstrates that manipulating children's phonological skills before reading instruction begins influences children's eventual reading ability. This therefore shows that phonological skills do have a causal role in reading development.

A number of people have argued that the reverse relationship also holds and that reading ability has a key role in developing phonemic awareness and phonemic processing skills (see Morais 1991, for an overview). The basis for this argument is that phonemes are rather abstract (even artificial) categories which correspond to a range of different perceptual experiences. For example, the /t/ in tin has quite different perceptual features from the /t/ in cotton. Although children may acquire knowledge of phonemes without reading experience (Content *et al.*, 1982; Lundberg *et al.*, 1988) it is clear that learning about words' spellings can facilitate the acquisition of phonemic knowledge (Perfetti *et al.*, 1987). Perfetti *et al.* (see also Goswami and Bryant, 1990; Wagner and Torgeson, 1987) have argued that reading and phonological skills influence one another interactively during development. We would therefore expect to find influences in both directions during development.

A slightly different type of training study has recently been reported by Hatcher, Hulme and Ellis (in press). They took as their starting point Bradley and Bryant's (1985) finding that integrated sound-categorisation and letter-knowledge training produced the largest improvements in reading and spelling. Their study was therefore designed to determine whether it was the integration of the two forms of knowledge that was important. Seven-year-old children who had failed to make the expected progress in reading were divided into four matched groups and assigned to a control condition or one of three experimental teaching conditions. The three experimental conditions were: reading with phonological skills training, reading alone, and phonological skills training alone. The group who received only phonological skills training showed the most improvement on phonological tasks but they did not make the most progress in reading. The most progress in reading was made by the group who received training in phonological skills together with reading instruction. This group also showed greater gains in reading than the group who received only (and hence more) reading instruction. This finding is interesting because it shows that success in reading is not related to the amount of phonological skills training nor to the amount of reading training; rather it is related to the integration of phonological and reading skills. A possible explanation for the greater success of this type of training is that it supports the bi-directional, reciprocal relationships between reading and phonological skills of the kind proposed by Perfetti (1985).

PROFILES OF READING ABILITIES IN DYSLEXIA

The argument that we have been developing has been concerned with the influence of phonological skills on reading processes. If this argument is to be fully developed, it is necessary to investigate the reading abilities – and difficulties – of dyslexic children and show how proposed deficits may give rise to the pattern of abilities that is observed. The phonological deficit hypothesis predicts that dyslexics should have problems in those aspects of reading that involve phonological processing. Phonological processes are required when unfamiliar words have to be decoded or 'sounded out'. Familiar words may be recognised more directly without the need to generate a sound-based representation. However, when reading aloud, a spoken form still has to be retrieved even if the process of recognition is visually based. A direct recognition process and 'sounding out' processes are widely recognised in most conceptualisations of reading systems although there is continued controversy as to the precise characterisation of each process (see van Orden, Pennington and Stone, 1990).

Phonological decoding skills can be measured most reliably by presenting 'nonsense words' which are novel letter strings that can be pronounced as if they were real words (e.g., *hin, lut, twamket* and *thringeld*). Direct recognition is often assessed by presenting irregular words such as island, gone and yacht which can only be pronounced correctly using more specific word knowledge. A number of studies have looked at the relative contributions of these two components of word reading skills to dyslexics' overall abilities. If dyslexics have a specific deficit in phonological processing, then we might expect their reading abilities to be made up more from the less-phonological, direct, component.

The largest study of component processes in dyslexics' word reading has been reported by Olson *et al.* (1989) who compared 172 dyslexic readers with a reading level-matched group of 172 normal readers. Subjects were given 85 one- and two-syllable nonwords to read and performance was assessed using a combination of accuracy and pronunciation latency data. The dyslexic readers were significantly worse than the younger normal readers; their average score was about three-quarters of a standard deviation below the mean for the normal group. In contrast, the dyslexic readers showed an advantage over their younger comparison group on a test of direct (or visual) recognition of words. In this task, subjects were asked to indicate which of two similar sounding letter strings was spelled correctly (e.g., salmon–sammon). Thus, when matched for overall reading level, the dyslexics showed a relatively greater reliance on the direct (or visual) processes for word recognition. This finding is therefore consistent with the phonological deficit hypothesis which states that dyslexics' difficulties will be most apparent when they have to use phonological processes.

A number of other studies have found dyslexics to show this same pattern of a deficiency in nonword reading when compared to reading level-matched normal readers (e.g., DiBenedetto, Richardson and Kochnower, 1983; Manis *et al.,* 1988; Siegel and Ryan, 1988; Snowling, 1980; 1981). However, other studies have found that dyslexics and reading level-matched normal readers have similar nonword reading abilities (e.g., Szeszulski and Manis, 1987; Treiman and Hirsh-Pasek, 1985; Vellutino and Scanlon, 1987). Reasons for the inconsistencies between these two sets of studies has been discussed extensively by Rack, Snowling and Olson (1992) who concluded that there were several possible reasons why studies might have failed to find a difference on nonword reading tasks. These included the use of nonwords that were too easy, difficulties with the tests used for matching the groups, and possible regression to the mean effects. However, all of the studies demonstrate the importance of phonological decoding skills for the successful development of reading abilities and the balance of the evidence suggests that phonological decoding deficits are likely to precede reading and spelling difficulties.

A related source of evidence comes from studying the nature of the reading errors made by dyslexics. Traditionally, dyslexics have been thought of as displaying visual incompetence – they 'see' words the wrong way round. Classic 'dyslexic' errors include reading *was* as *saw* (and vice versa) and *beard* as *bread,* as well as confusions over similar looking letters such as b and d, t and f. However, these errors are actually quite common in young children's reading at an early developmental stage (Seymour and MacGregor, 1984; Stuart and Coltheart 1988) and seem to be more closely associated with weak phonological skills. For example, Stuart and Coltheart found that subjects made a greater proportion of errors which preserved first and last letters sounds (and hence a lower proportion of 'visual' errors) at almost exactly the point in development when their phonological skills had become established. The common finding that dyslexics tend to make a large number of 'visual' reading errors (e.g., Olson *et al.*, 1985; Snowling, Stackhouse and Rack, 1986) is thus consistent with the view that they are not making use of phonological processes in reading to the same degree as do normally developing readers.

READING DEVELOPMENT

We come now to the most difficult part of our task, that of explaining how phonological deficits in memory and other verbal processes cause phonological deficits in word reading. In order to address this problem it is necessary to have a model of the process of reading development. Such a model is also needed in order to interpret the pattern of difficulties shown by dyslexics as was apparent in the discussion of reading errors (see Snowling, 1983; 1987 for further discussion). In addition, it is clear that disorder can only be interpreted relative to an established 'normal' pattern of development, furthermore, the pattern of difficulties is likely to change over time in a developmental disorder such as dyslexia. Summaries of three of the most influential models of reading development (Ehri, 1992; Frith, 1985; Marsh *et al.*, 1981) are given below. (For more discussion see Goswami and Bryant, 1990; Rack, Hulme and Snowling, 1993).

Marsh *et al.* (1981) divided reading development into four stages, Frith's (1985) model, which starts a little later in development, has only three stages. Marsh *et al.*'s first stage involves rote learning of frequently encountered words like a child's name, but unfamiliar words can only be guessed at using linguistic context. In Marsh *et al.*'s second stage, called discrimination net guessing, children begin to make use of visual features to discriminate between different words. Children will still guess at unfamiliar words using linguistic context but their guesses will share visual features with the target word. This stage is broadly similar to Frith's first stage, which is called logographic reading. In Marsh *et al.*'s third stage, called sequential decoding, children begin to decode unfamiliar words from left to right using simple grapheme–phoneme correspondence rules. At this stage only simple words comprising consonant-vowel-consonant (CVC) structures can be dealt with. This is very similar to Frith's second stage which is called alphabetic reading. Frith proposed that alphabetic reading involves decoding 'grapheme-by-grapheme' and that the shift to this kind of processing is brought about through spelling experience. Frith's final stage is the orthographic stage in which words are recognised in terms of orthographic units which, Frith states, should ideally coincide with morphemes. Orthographic strategies are distinguished from logographic strategies in that they involve analytic, abstract letter (not visual) processing. Unlike alphabetic strategies, orthographic strategies are non-phonological and involve larger units of words. Marsh *et al.*'s fourth stage seems to fit somewhere between alphabetic and orthographic reading. In this stage more complex, conditional or context-sensitive decoding rules are acquired and, it is proposed, analogy strategies are acquired.

Ehri's model has some similarities to Frith's and Marsh *et al.*'s models; however, it is primarily concerned with the way in which familiar words are recognised. Ehri proposed three phases in reading acquisition: visual cue reading, phonetic cue reading and phonemic map reading. Visual cue reading is very like discrimination net guessing and logographic reading; children make use of salient visual features of words, or features of the word's context, to access meanings. In Ehri's second phase children are thought to use phonetic cues for accessing word meanings. Children in this phase make use of the phonetic characteristics of words at a fairly basic level to help access pronunciations (and then meanings). A study by Ehri and Wilce (1985) showed that once children have some letter-sound knowledge, they are more likely to learn systematic nonwords (GRF for giraffe) than arbitrary nonwords (XBT for giraffe). These nonwords cannot be decoded by traditional grapheme–phoneme rules but, clearly, children do make use of the sounds of the letter string to help them form connections between the visual stimulus and the word's pronunciation. The third phase in Ehri's model involves a fully specified phonemic mapping of letters onto sounds. Readers in this phase make use of all the information in the word and are therefore less prone to the confusions that phase 2 readers would make. Ehri proposed that the reader in this phase is analysing the word down to the phonemic level in contrast to phase 2 readers who use phonetic cues that could be at any level from the syllable to the phoneme. A prerequisite for phonemic map phase is, therefore, the ability to segment speech sounds at the phonemic level. Ehri suggested that the transition between phases 2 and 3 may more accurately be thought of as gradual and quantitative rather than qualitative.

Dyslexia in the context of models of reading development

All the models of reading development discussed above include a stage in which phonological processes are very salient. These models can therefore accommodate the associations between phonological skills and reading ability observed in longitudinal studies and comparisons of good and poor readers. For example, Frith (1985; see also Snowling, 1987) proposed that dyslexics fail to make the transition from logographic to alphabetic reading because of problems with phoneme awareness and segmentation skill. The argument has been made that such a problem would have most impact on the development of phonological reading skills, but word-recognition abilities could still develop (using logographic skills) given enough exposure to printed words (Snowling, 1980; Olson *et al.*, 1985). Seymour (1986; 1990) argued that specific deficits can occur in both the alphabetic system and the orthographic system and that each of these deficits gives rise to different types of dyslexia. However, the evidence to show that *specific* orthographic difficulties can be caused by non-phonological factors has yet to be produced.

Ehri's model of reading acquisition suggests that phonological processes are important in the very earliest stages of sight-word development. Dyslexics may therefore have difficulties even with the early word learning that previously has been thought to be visually based. Before pursuing this idea, however, there are some limitations in Ehri and Wilce's (1985) study that need to be addressed. To do so, some data from a pilot study are reported next in which Ehri and Wilce's findings are clarified and extended.

The use of phonetic cues in early word learning

Ehri and Wilce (1985) taught children to associate letter strings (or cues) with spoken words (targets) in a paired-associate learning task. They compared children's performance on two types of cue. The phonetic cues (*GRF*, *LFNT*) contained letters whose sounds were present in the target words (*giraffe* and *elephant*), whereas the visual cues (*XbT*) were selected to be visually distinctive and discriminable. Pre-readers did better with the visually distinctive cues but, once they had letter sound knowledge, beginning readers did better with the phonetic cues.

One potential problem with Ehri and Wilce's study concerns the nature of the information which enabled some children to benefit from the 'phonetic cues'. Ehri and Wilce propose that *GRF* served as a successful cue to *giraffe* because children extracted the letter-names (*'jee are eff'*) which then cued a phonological representation of the word. However, children may have seen the written form of *giraffe* on previous occasions and the cue *GRF* could then serve to access (albeit incomplete) orthographic representations. In short, we cannot be sure that the phonetic cues were more successful because of their greater phonological or their greater visual similarity to the corresponding word form.

In a recent pilot study by the author, phonetic cues and control cues were selected so that they had an equal numbers of letters that were present in the word's spelling and they therefore looked like the target word's spelling to the same degree. The critical difference between the two types of cue occurred on a single letter which did not occur in the word's spelling. For the phonetic cues the sound of this letter was very similar to one in the target word, differing only in the articulatory feature of voicing. So, for example the phonetic cue for *table* was *dbl* the phonetic cue for *river* was *rfr*. In the control cues, there was a single letter whose sound was unrelated, or at least less similar, to a sound in the target word. Hence the control cue for *table* was *kbl* and the control cue for *river* was *rzr*. Any benefit of *dbl* over *kbl* has to come from the fact that the sound made by the letter *d* is phonetically similar to the sound made by the letter *t*; it cannot arise because of any greater visual overlap between *dbl* and *table* compared to *kbl* and *table*.

The experiment was also designed to investigate the effects of the position of cues within words. It is often reported that the first letter in the word is particularly salient so misreadings of words tend to contain the first letter of the intended word (e.g., Stuart and Coltheart, 1988). In half the cues in the present study the phonetic/control distinction was created by changing a letter in the middle of the word, leaving the first letter as 'correct' (e.g., *pgt* or *pft* for *packet*). In the other cues, the distinction was made by changing the first letter (e.g., *dbl* or *kbl* for *table*). On the basis of previous findings it might be predicted that children would do better with the cues where the change was made in the middle of the letter string.

Sixteen subjects took part in this study, their mean age being 4.9 years. They were given eight words to learn to associate with four different types of cue (phonetic and control cues in either beginning or middle positions). Two versions of the experiment were made so that every word was paired once with a phonetic cue and once with a control cue. Any differences in learning could not therefore be due to general differences in learning particular words. The words used were all bisyllabic and were chosen to be within the spoken vocabularies but not the written vocabularies of the subjects. Five teach-test trials were given and the number of words learned at the end of that period was taken as a dependent measure.

Subjects learned more of the words that were paired with phonetic cues and they learned more of the words in which the letter-change had been made in the middle. The means (and standard deviations) for the four conditions were as follows: Phonetic Cue, Middle (e.g., pgt–packet) 1.38 (0.62); Phonetic Cue, Beginning (e.g., dbl–table) 0.87 (0.62); Control Cue Middle (e.g., pft–packet) 0.88 (0.89); Control Cue, Beginning (e.g., kbl–table) 0.63 (0.72).

Repeated measures analysis of variance revealed significant effects of phonetic similarity [$F(1,15) = 5.00$, $p < .05$] and position [$F(1,15) = 9.00$, $p < .01$], with no interaction. This analysis indicates that the phonetic cues were more effective than the control cues even though these two types of cue were equally similar to the target word in terms of their spellings. The cues whose first letter was present in the word's spelling were more effective than the cues in which the first letter had been changed to a different (phonetic or control) letter.

These results suggest that children do make use of the sound-properties of words when they are committing them to a sight vocabulary. However, they do this in a very implicit fashion making use of phonetic (sound-property) information rather than phonemic (sound-identity) information. Indeed, the children in the present study were unable to read simple CVC nonwords, confirming that they would not be regarded as alphabetic readers. The present results therefore support the contention of Ehri (1992) that early 'logographic' reading may well be influenced by phonological factors. These results are only preliminary and they are limited by the small numbers of items used. However, the effect has now been replicated in a more extensive study (see Rack *et al.*, 1994).

Phonological difficulties reconsidered

Studies such as Ehri and Wilce's (1985) and the one reported here have led to the view that phonological processes are involved in the earliest stages of learning to read – as soon as children know some of the letters of the alphabet. Dyslexic readers, who are phonologically deficient, may therefore encounter problems from the earliest stages of development. However, since dyslexics are able to acquire letter-sound knowledge – even if they do so more slowly – they could make use of phonetic features of words to access pronunciations and meanings even if they have difficulty with the more complex processes of grapheme–phoneme decoding. Recall that in the pilot study reported here young children could use phonetic cues in word-learning but could not decode simple nonwords. Thus, dyslexics make more limited use of phonetic cues during reading, but would not 'read without phonology' as some have suggested.

This extension of Ehri's model has some interesting implications for considering individual differences in dyslexia: different degrees of phonological deficit would become restrictive at different points in the development of phonetic-cue and phonemic-map reading. Olson *et al.* (1985) suggested that dyslexics may differ in terms of the level of segmentation that their phonological skills would support. Coarse phonological segmentation might therefore permit phonetic-cue reading but would prevent progress to phonemic-map reading. Thus the extension of Ehri's model provides a theoretical basis for the observed relationship between segmental language skills and reading development.

CONCLUSIONS

The objective for deficit accounts of dyslexia is to explain how difficulties in processing outside the domain of reading impact upon the development of reading skills. In the present chapter, we have seen that many of the components of such an explanation are now available. It seems clear that dyslexics tend to have difficulties in a variety of verbal memory tasks which require access to a sound-based code. Dyslexics' difficulties seem to be especially pronounced when they have to process small units of sounds such as phonemes. A number of longitudinal studies have shown that these phonological abilities are related to reading ability. Furthermore, improving phonological skills produces consequent improvements in reading and spelling (Bradley and Bryant, 1985; Lundberg *et al.*, 1988; Hatcher, Hulme and Ellis in press). We have also seen that dyslexics have difficulty reading nonsense words and that their errors often indicate a more 'visual' approach to word recognition.

Learning experiments such as the one reported in the present chapter can offer some insights into the connections between phonological deficits in verbal memory and reading difficulties. In the phonetic cue experiment children learned to recognise strings of letters which is, of course, what happens when new words are learned. Even though the letter strings could not be 'decoded', phonetic information was extracted from them and this was used to help commit them to memory. However, the letter strings did eventually become quite familiar suggesting that the child was also building up a visual representation in memory. We might reasonably ask how phonetic cues help to establish these visual representations. One possible sequence of events is described below. If nothing else, this may serve to remind us that there is still more work to be done in order to understand the role of phonological skills in dyslexia.

When the child sees a written word, letter-sound information is extracted from the word string (initially, this may be confined to the first letter or the first and last letters). At the same time there is a process of visual access by which (partial) visual representations, formed on previous exposures, are accessed. In this way, visually similar items are likely to be activated and, at least in the early stages of learning, there may be no clear 'winner' to be recognised. Phonological information associated with the visual representations (again partial) may then be retrieved. This information may then converge with phonological information derived from letter-sound processes and, where there is an overlap, the associations between the visual letter string, the visual representation and the stored spoken form become strengthened. In the later stages of learning, the process could be very similar except that letter strings could (as connections become strengthened) access their corresponding visual and spoken representations more specifically.

The operation of these processes depends upon: (1) having letter-sound knowledge; (2) access to representations of previously seen words; (3) retrieval of associated phonological information; (4) maintenance of two sources of phonological information in a working memory system; and, (5) ability to register (implicitly) similarities between different sources of phonological information. As we saw in the first part of this chapter, dyslexics would be expected to have difficulties with at least three of these five processes. If this type of explanation could be substantiated with further research we would have made considerable progress towards an information processing-based understanding of developmental dyslexia.

Finally, let us consider whether the definition of dyslexia should be altered to reflect the progress that has been made towards this goal. There are several reasons to be cautious. Open questions remain about the origins of a phonological deficit, specifically whether it might relate to an earlier deficit in syntactic processing (Scarborough, 1991). Another unresolved area concerns individual differences. In the present chapter we have considered group studies which give us generalisable information about *most* people. Interpretation of individual differences in a developmental context is very difficult and, as yet, we do not know whether specific deficits in other processing skills might be found. We would not want to restrict a definition of dyslexia, at this stage, to one of a phonological disorder. However, it is quite clear that phonological skills play a central role in the majority of dyslexics' difficulties.

REFERENCES

Baddeley, A.D. (1966). Short–term memory for word sequences as a function of acoustic semantic and formal similarity. *Quarterly Journal of Experimental Psychology, 18,* 262–265.

Baddeley, A.D. (1986). *Working Memory.* Oxford: Oxford University Press.

Boder, E.M. (1973). Developmental dyslexia: A diagnostic approach based on three atypical reading–spelling patterns. *Developmental Medicine and Child Neurology, 15,* 663–687.

Bauer, R.H. and Emhert, J. (1984). Information processing in reading disabled and nondisabled readers. *Journal of Experimental Child Psychology, 37,* 271–281.

Bradley, L.L. and Bryant, P. (1978). Difficulties in auditory organization as a possible cause of reading backwardness. *Nature, 271,* 746–747.

Bradley, L.L. and Bryant, P.E. (1983). Categorizing sounds and learning to read: A causal connexion. *Nature, 301,* 419.

Bradley, L.L. and Bryant, P.E. (1985). *Rhyme and Reason in Reading and Spelling.* Ann Arbor: University of Michigan Press.

Brady, S. (1986). Short-term memory, phonological processing and reading ability. *Annals of Dyslexia, 36,* 138–153.

Bryant, P.E., and Goswami, U.C. (1987). Phonological awareness and learning to read. In J. Beech and A. Colley (Eds.) *Cognitive Approaches to Reading.* (pp. 163–178). Chichester: Wiley.

Byrne, B. and Shea, P. (1979). Semantic and phonetic memory codes in beginning readers. *Memory and Cognition, 7,* 333–338.

Cataldo, S. and Ellis, N.C. (1990). Learning to spell, learning to read. In P.D. Pumfrey and C.D. Elliot (Eds.) *Children's Difficulties in Reading, Spelling and Writing.* Basingstoke: Falmer Press.

Catts, H.W. (1989). Defining dyslexia as a developmental language disorder. *Annals of Dyslexia, 39,* 50–64.

Cohen, R.L. and Netley, C. (1981). Short–term memory deficits in reading disabled children in the absence of opportunities for rehearsal strategies. *Intelligence, 5,* 69–76.

Conners, F.A. and Olson, R.K. (1990). Reading comprehension in dyslexic and normal readers: A component skills analysis. In D.A. Balota, G.B. Flores d'Arcais and K. Rayner (Eds.), *Comprehension Processes in Reading* (pp. 1–23). Hillsdale, NJ: Erlbaum.

Conrad, R. (1964). Acoustic confusions in immediate memory. *British Journal of Psychology, 55,* 75–84.

Content, A., Morais, J., Alegria, J. and Bertelson, P. (1982). Accelerating the development of phonemic segmentation skills in kindergartners. *Cahiers de Psychologie Cognitive, 2,* 259-269.

Critchley, M. (1970). *The Dyslexic Child.* London: Heinemann Medical Books.

DiBenedetto, B., Richardson, E. and Kochnower, J. (1983). Vowel generation in normal and learning disabled readers. *Journal of Educational Psychology, 75,* 576–582.

Ehri, L.C. (1987). Learning to read and spell words. *Journal of Reading Behaviour, 19,* 5–31.

Ehri, L.C. (1989). The development of spelling knowledge and its role in reading acquisition and reading disability. *Journal of Learning Disabilities, 22,* 356–365.

Ehri, L.C. (1992). Reconceptualizing the development of sight-word reading and its relationship to decoding. In P.B. Gough, L.C. Ehri, and R. Treiman (Eds.), *Reading Acquisition.* London: Lawrence Erlbaum.

Ehri, L., and Wilce, L.S. (1980). The influence of orthography on readers' conceptualization of the phonemic structure of words. *Applied Psycholinguistics, 1,* 371–385

Ehri, L.C. and Wilce, L.S. (1985). Movement into reading: Is the first stage of printed word learning visual or phonetic? *Reading Research Quarterly, 20,* 163–179.

Ehri, L.C. and Wilce, L.S. (1987). Cipher versus cue reading: An experiment in decoding acquisition. *Journal of Educational Psychology, 79,* 3–13.

Ellis, N.C. (1991). Spelling and sound in learning to read. In M.J. Snowling and M. Thompson (Eds.), *Dyslexia: Integrating Theory and Practice* (pp. 80–94). London: Whurr.

Fletcher, J.M. and Morris, R. (1986). Classification of disabled readers: Beyond exclusionary definition. In S.J. Ceci (Ed.), *Handbook of Cognitive, Social and Neuropsychological Aspects of Learning Difficulties* (pp. 55–80). Hillsdale, NJ: Erlbaum

Frick, R.W. (1984). Using both an auditory and a visual short–term store to increase digit span. *Memory and Cognition, 12,* 507–514.

Frith, U. (1981). Experimental approaches to developmental dyslexia: An introduction. *Psychological Research, 43,* 97–109.

Frith, U. (1985). Beneath the surface of developmental dyslexia. In K.E. Patterson, J.C. Marshall, and M. Coltheart (Eds.), *Surface Dyslexia.* London: Routledge and Kegan Paul.

Gathercole, S.E. and Baddeley, A.D. (1989). Evaluation of the role of phonological STM in the development of vocabulary in children: A longitudinal study. *Journal of Memory and Language, 28,* 200–213.

Gleitman, L.R. and Rozin, P. (1977). The structure and acquisition of reading I: Relations between orthographies and the structure of language. In R.S. Reber and D.L. Scarborough (Eds.), *Toward a Psychology of Reading* (pp. 1–54). Hillsdale, NJ: Erlbaum.

Goswami, U. and Bryant, P.E. (1990). *Phonological Skills and Learning to*

Read. London: LEA.

Hall, J., Wilson, K., Humphreys, M., Tinzman, M. and Bowyer, P. (1983). Phonemic similarity effects in good versus poor readers. *Memory and Cognition, 11*, 520–527.

Hatcher, P., Hulme, C. & Ellis, A.W. (1994, in press). Ameliorating early reading failure by integrating the teaching of reading and phonological skills. *Child Development*.

Holligan, C., and Johnston, R. (1988). The use of phonological information by good and poor readers in memory and reading tasks. *Memory and Cognition, 16*, 522–532.

Hulme, C. and Snowling, M. (1991). Phonological deficits in dyslexia: A 'sound' reappraisal of the verbal deficit hypothesis? In N. Singh and I. Beale (Eds.), *Progress in Learning Disabilities*. Berlin: Springer-Verlag.

Johnston, R., Rugg, M. and Scott, T. (1987). Phonological similarity effects, memory span and developmental reading disorders: The nature of the relationship. *British Journal of Psychology, 78*, 205–211.

Jorm, A.F., Share, D.L., MacLean, R. and Matthews, R. (1984). Phonological confusability in short–term memory for sentences as a predictor of reading ability. *British Journal of Psychology, 75*, 393–400.

Katz, R. (1986). Phonological deficiencies in children with reading disability: Evidence from an object naming task. *Cognition, 22*, 225–257.

Liberman, A.M. and Shankweiler, D.P. (1979). Speech, the alphabet and teaching to read. In L. Resnick and P. Weaver (Eds.), *Theory and Practice of Early Reading*. Hillsdale, NJ: Lawrence Erlbaum Associates.

Liberman, I.Y., Shankweiler, D., Fischer, W.F., and Carter, B. (1974). Reading and the awareness of linguistic segments. *Journal of Experimental Child Psychology, 18,* 201–212.

Lundberg, I., Olofson, A. and Wall, S. (1980). Reading and spelling skills in the first school years predicted from phonemic awareness skills in kindergarten. *Scandinavian Journal of Psychology, 21*, 159–173.

Lundberg, I., Frost, J. and Peterson, O. (1988). Effects of an extensive program for stimulating phonological awareness in preschool children. *Reading Research Quarterly, 23*, 263–284.

Manis, F.R., Szeszulski, P.A., Holt, L.K. and Graves, K. (1988). A developmental perspective on dyslexic subtypes. *Annals of Dyslexia, 38*, 139–153.

Mann, V.A. (1984). Reading skill and language skill. *Developmental Review, 4*, 1–15.

Mann, V. and Liberman, I.Y. (1984). Phonological awareness and verbal short–term memory: Can they presage early reading success? *Journal of Learning Disabilities, 17*, 592–599.

Mark, L.S., Shankweiler, D., Liberman, I. and Fowler, C. (1977). Phonetic recoding in the beginning reader. *Memory and Cognition, 5*, 623–629.

Marsh, G., Friedman, M., Welch, V., and Desberg, P. (1981). A cognitive–developmental theory of reading acquisition. In G.E. MacKinnon and T.G. Waller (Eds.), *Reading Research: Advances in theory and practice* (Vol. 3). New York: Academic Press.

Miles, T.R. (1983). *Dyslexia: The pattern of difficulties.* Oxford: Blackwell. 2nd edition, 1993, London: Whurr.

Morais, J. (1991). Metaphonological abilities and literacy. In M. J. Snowling and M. Thompson (Eds.), *Dyslexia: Integrating theory and practice* (pp. 95–107). London: Whurr.

Morrison, F.J. and Manis, F.R. (1983). Cognitive processes in reading disability: a critique and proposal. In C.J. Brainerd and M. Pressley (Eds.), *Progress in Cognitive Development Research.* New York: Springer–Verlag.

Olson, R.K., Kliegel, R., Davidson, B.J. and Davies, S.E. (1984). Development of phonetic memory in disabled and normal readers. *Journal of Experimental Child Psychology, 37*, 187–206.

Olson, R.K., Davidson, B.J., Kliegel, R., and Foltz, G. (1985). Individual and developmental differences in reading disability. In G.E. MacKinnon and T.G. Waller (Eds.), *Reading Research: Advances in theory and practice* (Vol. 4, pp. 1–64). New York: Academic Press.

Olson, R.K., Rack, J.P. and Forsberg, H. (1990). Profiles of abilities in dyslexics and reading–level–matched controls. Poster presented at the Rodin Remediation Academy meeting at Boulder, Colorado, September 1990.

Olson, R.K., Wise, B., Conners, F., Rack, J., and Fulker, D. (1989). Specific deficits in component reading and language skills: Genetic and environmental influences. *Journal of Learning Disabilities, 22*, 339–348.

Olson, R.K., Wise, B., Conners, F.A., and Rack, J.P. (1990). Organization, heritability, and remediation of component word recognition and language skills in disabled readers. In T.H. Carr and B.A. Levy (Eds.), *Reading and its Development: Component skills approaches* (pp. 261–322). New York: Academic Press.

Olson, R.K., Gillis, J.J., Rack, J.P., DeFries, J.C. and Fulker, D.W. (1991). Confirmatory factor analysis of word recognition and process measures in the Colorado reading project. *Reading and Writing, 3,* 235–248.

Perfetti, C. (1985). *Reading Ability.* New York: Oxford University Press.

Perfetti, C.A., Beck, I., Bell, L.C., and Hughes, C. (1987). Phonemic knowledge and learning to read are reciprocal: A longitudinal study of first grade children. *Merrill Palmer Quarterly, 33*, 283–319.

Rack, J. (1985). Orthographic and phonetic coding in normal and dyslexic readers. *British Journal of Psychology, 76*, 325–340.

Rack, J.P. and Snowling M.J. (1985). Verbal deficits in dyslexia: A review. In M.J. Snowling (Ed.), *Children's Written Language Difficulties: Assessment and management.* Windsor: NFER-Nelson.

Rack, J.P., Hulme, C. and Snowling, M.J. (1993). Learning to read: A theoretical synthesis. In H. Reese (Ed.), *Advances in Child Development and Behaviour*. Vol. 24. New York: Academic Press.

Rack, J.P., Hulme, C., Snowling, M.J. and Wightman, J. (1994). The role of phonology in young children's learning of sight words: The direct mapping hypothesis. *Journal of Experimental Child Psychology, 57*, 42–71.

Rack, J.P., Snowling, M.J. and Olson, R.K. (1992). The nonword reading deficit in developmental dyslexia: A review. *Reading Research Quarterly, 27*, 28–53.

Rozin, P. and Gleitman, L.R. (1977). The structure and acquisition of reading II: The reading process and the acquisition of the alphabetic principle. In R.S. Reber and D.L. Scarborough (Eds.), *Toward a Psychology of Reading* (pp. 55–141). Hillsdale, NJ: Erlbaum

Rugel, R.P. (1974). WISC subtest scores of disabled readers: A review with respect to Bannatyne's recategorization. *Journal of Learning Disabilities, 7*, 48–55.

Scarborough, H.S. (1991). Very early language deficits in dyslexic children. *Child Development, 61*, 1728–1743.

Seymour, P.H.K. (1986). *Cognitive Analysis of Dyslexia*. London: Routledge and Kegan Paul.

Seymour, P.H.K. (1990). Developmental dyslexia. In M.W. Eysenck (Ed.), *Cognitive Psychology: An international review* (pp. 135–196). Chichester: John Wiley.

Seymour, P.H.K. and Elder, L. (1986). Beginning reading without phonology. *Cognitive Neuropsychology, 3*, 1–36.

Seymour, P.H.K. and MacGregor, C.J. (1984). Developmental dyslexia: A cognitive developmental analysis of phonological morphemic and visual impairments. *Cognitive Neuropsychology, 1*, 43–82.

Shankweiler, D. and Liberman, I.Y. (1990). *Phonology and Reading Disability: Solving the reading puzzle*. Ann Arbor: University of Michigan Press.

Shankweiler, D., Liberman, I.Y., Mark, L.S., Fowler, C.A. and Fischer, F.W. (1979). The speech code and learning to read. *Journal of Experimental Psychology: Human learning and memory, 5*, 531–545.

Siegel, L.S. (1988). Evidence that IQ scores are irrelevant to the definition and analysis of reading disability. *Canadian Journal of Psychology, 42*, 201–215.

Siegel, L.S. and Linder, B.A. (1984). Short-term memory processes in children with reading and arithmetic learning disabilities. *Developmental Psychology, 20*, 200–207.

Siegel, L.S. and Ryan, E.B. (1988). Development of grammatical–sensitivity, phonological, and short–term memory skills in normally achieving and learning disabled children. *Developmental Psychology, 24*, 28–37.

Snowling, M.J. (1980). The development of grapheme–phoneme correspondences in normal and dyslexic readers. *Journal of Experimental Child Psychology, 29,* 294–305.

Snowling, M.J. (1981). Phonemic deficits in developmental dyslexia. *Psychological Research, 43,* 219–234.

Snowling, M.J. (1983). The comparison of acquired and developmental disorders of reading. *Cognition, 14,* 105–118.

Snowling, M. (1987). *Dyslexia: A cognitive developmental perspective.* Blackwell: Oxford.

Snowling, M.J., Goulandris, N., Bowlby, M. and Howell, P. (1986). Segmentation and speech perception in relation to reading skill: A developmental analysis. *Journal of Experimental Child Psychology, 41,* 489–507.

Snowling, M.J., Stackhouse, R.J. and Rack, J.P. (1986). Phonological dyslexia and dysgraphia – a developmental analysis. *Cognitive Neuropsychology, 3,* 309–339.

Snowling, M., van Wagtendonk, B. and Stafford, C. (1988). Object–naming deficits in developmental dyslexia. *Journal of Research in Reading, 11,* 67–85.

Stanovich, K.E. (1986). Cognitive processes and the reading problems of learning disabled children: Evaluating the assumption of specificity. In J.K. Torgesen and B.Y.L. Wong (Eds.), *Psychological and Educational Perspectives on Learning Disabilities.* Orlando, FL: Academic Press.

Stanovich, K.E. (1988). Explaining the differences between the dyslexic and the garden-variety poor reader: The phonological-core variable-difference model. *Journal of Learning Disabilities, 21,* 590–612.

Stanovich, K.E., Cunningham, A.E. and Cramer, B.B. (1984). Assessing phonological skills in kindergarten children: Issues of task comparability. *Journal of Experimental Child Psychology, 38,* 175–190

Sternberg, R.J. (Ed.), (1982). *Handbook of Human Intelligence.* Cambridge: Cambridge University Press.

Stuart, M. and Coltheart, M. (1988). Does reading develop in a sequence of stages? *Cognition, 30,* 139–181.

Szeszulski, P. and Manis, F. (1987). A comparison of word recognition processes in dyslexic and normal readers at two different reading age levels. *Journal of Experimental Child Psychology, 44,* 364–376.

Taylor, H.G., Satz, P. and Friel, J. (1979). Developmental dyslexia in relation to other childhood disorders: Significance and utility. *Reading Research Quarterly, 15,* 84–101.

Treiman, R. and Hirsch-Pasek, K. (1985). Are there qualitative differences in reading behavior between dyslexic and normal readers? *Memory and Cognition, 13,* 357–364.

Van Orden, G.C., Pennington, B.F. and Stone, G.O. (1990). Word identification in reading and the promise of subsymbolic psycholinguistics. *Psychological Review, 97,* 488–522.

Vellutino, F.R. (1979). *Dyslexia: Theory and research.* Cambridge, MA: MIT Press.

Vellutino, F.R. and Scanlon, D.M. (1987). Phonological coding, phonological awareness, and reading ability: Evidence from a longitudinal and experimental study. *Merrill Palmer Quarterly, 33,* 321–364.

Wagner, R.K. and Torgesen, J.K. (1987). The nature of phonological processing and its casual role in the acquisition of reading skills. *Psychological Bulletin, 101,* 192–212.

Yopp, H.K. (1988). The reliability and validity of phonemic awareness tests. *Reading Research Quarterly, 23,* 159–177.

CHAPTER 2

Reading skills, strategies and their degree of tractability in dyslexia

John R. Beech

The term dyslexia means that a child or adult in this condition is considerably below normal reading age, is normal in intelligence, has no visual or auditory defects, is emotionally stable and has a normal educational opportunity. In effect, the definition is trying to eliminate possible problems that could have produced reading difficulties, apart from cognitive ones unrelated to general intelligence. In addition, it means that dyslexia cannot be diagnosed until some considerable time after beginning to learn to read. The definition is shrouded in controversy, especially the part about normal educational opportunity. Many who use the term dyslexia believe that this excludes those of low socioeconomic status as this may be a further reason for poor reading levels. The evidence supports such a connection. One problem is perhaps more political in that the definition excludes a proportion of poor readers who may as a consequence get neglected if resources are concentrated only on those with dyslexia. Another aspect is that giving a medical label of dyslexia may discourage the child from even trying; others argue that it actually brings a sense of relief and helps in the longer term. From a research viewpoint there is the advantage that this is a defined subject population which is relatively immutable. But many unresolved problems remain, such as: what exactly do we mean by 'controlling for intelligence', for instance, surely there are several cognitive processes (e.g., vocabulary, phonology) that are linked both to reading and to intelligence? How does socioeconomic status produce an effect on reading? Stanovich (1986) discusses these and other issues extensively.

Children with dyslexia can have problems with their reading for a variety of reasons. For example, they may have a more generalised problem in achieving automaticity in learning in general (Nicolson and Fawcett, 1990) or they may have problems in one or more potential routes or methods of reading. There are several potential types of skill for reading. The first that we shall examine is that involving translating a visual representation to a semantic one. This is sometimes referred to as an 'addressed phonology', implying that there is an addressed location from which the whole phonological code of a word may be retrieved. The visual representation evokes the meaning which enables retrieval by accessing the address of a stored phonological representation of that meaning. The processes involved here will be termed 'lexical', indicating that they derive from accessing the whole word.

The second type of skill or route is the segmentation of the letters into their graphemes (e.g., *ch*) from which phonemes are derived. These are blended to produce a code. Further refinements (e.g., Patterson and Morton, 1985) have suggested larger units than the grapheme, so instead of referring to grapheme–phoneme conversion, the term 'sublexical' processes will be used instead to encompass this possibility. This route has also been referred to as 'assembled phonology' due to the need to build up units of sound in an attempt to generate the appropriate word.

A final possibility is the activation of phonology directly from the visual representation without the activation of a semantic representation and without the activation of the sublexical route. There has only been one such case reported and this was a temporary aberration only (Schwartz, Saffran and Marin, 1980). However, we shall also examine a connectionist simulation of such a route.

The first two types of skill (lexical and sublexical) have had a dominating influence over theorising, especially in relation to the acquired dyslexias. Part of this theoretical structure has been the almost implicit assumption that if a child with dyslexia has problems in one route, the other route can be used to compensate this problem. But relying on just one route may be dysfunctional. We shall first examine the two major routes in detail and then examine this reciprocity assumption. We shall also examine more recent developments that have challenged dual-route theory along the way.

DEVELOPMENT OF LOGOGRAPHIC OR LEXICAL SKILLS

We shall now examine the development of the route involving the direct translation of a visual representation of a word to a semantic one. Initially this appears to be a very primitive process, but it develops later into an impressively fast process when the reader has become skilled. The initial process has been called 'logographic' processing.

The well-cited stage theorists of reading such as Frith (1985) and Marsh *et al.* (1981) have proposed that an early stage of reading involves the coding of a word as a collection of visual features. These features are then associated with their corresponding meaning. This method of reading poses the problem of differentiating different types of word patterns from each other for the reader; to overcome this some form of feature discrimination process is required. But this means that only a minimal set of visual features is stored, sufficient to distinguish a stored logographic configuration from other such representations. Seymour and Elder (1986) examined beginning readers taught without phonology, and demonstrated that their reading was likely to be featural rather than Gestalt-like. In other words, rather than a holistic representation minimising the impact of small detail (the sort one might see with eyes screwed up), the child codes the visual characteristics of the individual letters. As the numbers of such featural representations increase, further discriminations have to be made to differentiate new words from existing ones. Thus eventually, earlier learned words will consist of substantially more visual features than they did in the early stages.

Logographic processing is like the reading process of the

Chinese in which each representation of the word holds little or no clue to the sound accompanying that word. The retrieval of the meaning of the word and its subsequent sound is accomplished by accessing what is already stored about the print. The word *may* be identified by extracting a subset consisting of a sequence of letters and linking it to similar words, but that would be a different form of processing.

Logographic processing is considered to be a primitive form of processing that is the rudimentary beginning of the lexical route. It is not very clear how this route develops over time. Dual coding theorists (e.g., Coltheart, 1978) would argue that it is increasingly aided by a sublexical route, especially one involving letter-sound translation. However, after a further period of time the sublexical route is no longer normally used to identify the words. This has been called the 'by-pass' hypothesis (van Orden, Pennington and Stone, 1990).

The position of Stuart and Coltheart (1988) should also be noted; they emphasise the interactive nature of logographic and phonological reading from the earliest stage of reading. Children with initial phonological skills will deploy these in learning to read while others will be logographic.

Is logographic/lexical processing sustainable?

There is a general consensus that the primitive logographic route is insufficient in itself to sustain readers to achieve eventual maturity. Or to shift view slightly, the use of a sublexical route is considered to be important for reading. For instance, Hulme and Snowling (1992) state: 'some indirect route involving the translation of letters into sounds is certainly important in learning to read' (p. 67); Rayner and Pollatsek (1989) write: 'successful reading requires some awareness and mastery of the alphabetic principle' (p. 354). One could find many quotes on this point, ranging in position from the view that a sublexical route is essential to one suggesting that it is important.

There is some evidence that at first glance appears to lend weight to the view that sublexical processing is essential. Consider, for example, the progress of the hearing impaired reader, who (if the impairment is prelingual) has no access to a phonological code that could assist a sublexical route. Very few of them develop into mature readers, with only 1% achieving reading age level by the time they are 16 years (Gaines, Mandler and Bryant, 1981).

Recent work by Beech and Harris (1994) has demonstrated that such readers, by the time they have struggled to reach a reading age of 7 years, have a very impoverished sublexical route compared to a group of younger hearing readers who are reading normally for their age, matched to these hearing impaired readers with severe or profound levels of deafness. The hearing impaired were not affected by reading irregular words, which generate erroneous phonological codes (e.g., *yacht* rhymes with *hatched* if pronounced according to its spelling, which is very different from *yot*, the way it should be sounded). On the other hand, the hearing children were affected relative to reading regular words. Similarly, the hearing children made more errors rejecting homophonic nonwords (e.g., *werd*) compared with non-homophonous nonwords (e.g., *liston*) in a lexical decision task requiring them to accept words and reject nonwords; by contrast the hearing impaired were again unaffected. We have argued on the basis of these results that the hearing impaired children are continuing to expand their stored reading knowledge of words by means of logographic processes in the absence of a sublexical structure. This argument should be tempered by adding that it is likely that hearing impaired children also have problems in language development, especially if they are using signing, which has a grammatical structure that deviates from that of written and spoken language (e.g., Harris and Coltheart, 1986).

Impoverished comprehension could be a retarding influence in that the deaf readers' continuing exposure to print, and hence reading lexicon development, is diminished relative to hearing readers. This is why it is not so straightforward to argue that exclusive use of logographic skills would impair full development of reading in hearing children/adults with normal comprehension. This is a point we shall return to shortly.

Does logographic reading change qualitatively?

An interesting question to pose is whether the continuing development of reading under circumstances of impoverished phonology due to deafness still involves such a logographic process when the hearing impaired become maturer readers at their particular level. Or indeed, for any reader who relies on a purely logographic route, does the process change in a qualitative way? Perhaps there is a different type of processing of reading at that maturer stage? There are three strands of evidence that might suggest that the process could be the same. The first comes from connectionist simulations of reading suggesting that simple frequency of exposure to print could determine reading performance. The second comes from a case study of an apparently normal fluent reader who appears to have a severely impoverished sublexical route. Presumably she started out as a logographic reader and developed into a fluent reader without phonology assisting her in this development. The third aspect comes from work on the development of automaticity in normal reading.

Connectionist simulations of reading
The development of connectionist modelling techniques has led to considerable debate as to the appropriateness of the dual route model for word recognition. It should be stated at the outset with regard to the connectionist evidence that this is based on simulations in a very restricted domain, and the simulation was not actually on a logographic process (as previously defined) for two reasons. First, no actual lexical store of information was involved (but this point is debatable). Second, this particular simulation involved the connections of orthographic strings to phonological representations rather than semantic ones. Nevertheless, it is an innovative model that can show the potential of frequency of exposure of print as a mediating variable to explain several phenomena of reading derived from classical cognitive psychology.

The model in question is that of Seidenberg and McClelland (1989) (see also Patterson, Seidenberg and McClelland, 1989). It consists of three components: orthographic units, phonological units and hidden units. Taking these in turn, the orthographic units were based on units of strings of three adjacent letters, generated from each word; the phonological units were based on three adjacent phonemes within the word; and the hidden units were units which interconnect between the orthographic and phonological layers. Thus, the orthographic units connected to all the hidden units and all hidden units to the phonological units. The connections between the units carried weights that governed the spread of activation throughout the system. These weights encoded what the model 'knew' about the frequency and distribution of correspondences between orthography and phonology.

A corpus of words was presented to the system. Each word was stripped down into triples of adjacent characters, for instance, BAT would be *BA, BAT, AT* (the asterisk represents a space). The phonemes in each word were similarly coded as sets of triples. For example the word *bat* consists of three triples (or 'Wickelphones'): *ba, bat, at*. Each Wickelphone was encoded over a pattern of activation over a set of units representing phonetic features. Then the connection weights were set by a training sequence between the orthographic and phonological units, via the hidden units. This used a back-propagation algorithm. The weights were initially set randomly within a specified range.

Suppose one of the words in the corpus were *meat*. After a few cycles in which *meat* is presented, 20 or so orthographic units out of 400 will have a higher likelihood of activation as a result of learning. There will also be corresponding numbers of hidden and phonological units which will be activated.

An important aspect was that in each trial the probability of a word in the corpus being selected was determined by its frequency. This meant that a low-frequency word would be selected for relatively few trials, but a high-frequency word would be selected for virtually all the learning trials. Consequently the connections between high-frequency words and their corresponding phonological codes were the strongest, thus concurring with research into fluent and developing reading: high-frequency words are read faster.

Patterson *et al.* replicated a finding of Taraban and McClelland (1987) showing an interaction between word frequency and spelling regularity. This indicated that there are no differences in spelling regularity for high-frequency words, but at low frequencies irregularly spelled words are read more slowly than regularly spelled words.

Dual-route theory had proposed that the explanation for the distinction between regular and exception words was because exception words generate phonological codes (using grapheme–phoneme translation) that are different from the actual pronunciation of the word. But it had difficulty with interpreting the Taraban and McClelland result. By contrast, the connectionist model predicted the result and demonstrated that it could be produced entirely in terms of frequency of exposure of letter strings and their corresponding phonological representations. But the radical nature of the model is that it does not appear to have a lexicon.

To return to our original question, a connectionist model such as this, despite its potential faults (see Quinlan, 1991), does suggest that during the course of learning print, the processes involved (i.e., making connections between orthographic strings and some other mode of representation) are essentially the same. There is no need to invoke a stage model of reading development suggesting, for instance, the concept of passing from a logographic to an orthographic stage. The effect is that particular words eventually produce faster responses and fewer errors are committed.

Mature reading with minimal sublexical skill
The second part of the evidence that using the lexical route may be essentially the same process is provided by examining the case study of RE (Campbell and Butterworth, 1985).

RE was an undergraduate who could read fluently such irregular words as *placebo*, but had problems reading even simple nonwords. Thus she appears to have developed her reading entirely by logographic/lexical processing. By her own account she could only read aloud after hearing it being spoken. She had no history of speech or hearing difficulty. At school she had problems (from age 5 to 8) because phonic methods were tried and failed. Her mother taught her using the 'look-and-say' method. She then went to another school which used eclectic teaching methods. She passed the selection examination at 11 years and continued through the school system up to university. Thus she appears to have gained several years of reading age in a comparatively short space of time.

Campbell and Butterworth found that her verbal IQ was 123, but her digit span was 2 standard deviations below the mean for her age. Her reading and spelling performance were both good. In a list of 30 simple nonwords she pronounced 9 correctly, but she was very slow, taking 3 sec per item on average. When the words were longer she read 3 out of 20 correctly. When given word strings such as *mannerlaugh* she could read these without difficulty showing that the letter strings can be analysed into words. Her problem lay in breaking new strings into sublexical units, pronouncing them and then blending these pronunciations together. She found it difficult, but not impossible, to generate phonemes to presented letters.

Her reported phenomenological experience of reading as a silent activity is revealing. This concurs with her inability to decide if pairs of words rhymed when the spelling patterns looked different from one another (for example, *true/shoe*). This is likely to be a phenomenological characteristic of pure logographic/lexical reading in general: it is conducted silently.

Parenthetically, inner speech may have a reduced role while reading Chinese (Seidenberg, 1985) and selective interference by concurrent articulation has a greater effect on Kanji (in which characters represent syllables) than Kana (in which characters represent morphemes) in Japanese readers (Kimura and Bryant, 1983).

Thus RE is a reader who has developed a high level of reading skill without using a sublexical route, and who at a crucial stage of development had her mother at hand to supply her with the sounds of different words. Furthermore, she appears to have acquired her sight vocabulary very rapidly during this period. We do not have the advantage of having information on her reading in the early stages, but we might confidently suppose that, as in the connectionist model, the continued exposure to print led to eventual fluency. There were virtually no sublexical processes to interact with this development. When confronted with nonwords she did have a primitive knowledge of some letter-sound connections, but she appeared to use analogy more, in a slow, halting manner. Thus to return to the question of qualitative change in logographic reading, given that there appears to be little interaction with a sublexical route, there seems to have been no such change.

The development of automaticity

Horn and Manis (1987) report an experiment that gives a much more direct indication of the development of automaticity in normal reading development. They examined this development in readers from first to fifth grade and college students using a selective interference paradigm. The readers were given a semantic categorisation task in which two words were presented consecutively (e.g., *duck–cow*) and they responded whether they were in the same category, knowing that there were four possible categories (animals, colours, body parts and clothing). Randomly on half the trials they responded to a tone which occurred when the first word in the pair was presented. If this tone produced little or no interference, this was taken as an indication that the categorisation task could be undertaken automatically. However, if there was interference, this would indicate the extent to which the task was consuming resources. Horn and Manis found that interference effects were considerable at first grade, declined rapidly by second grade and then more slowly after that. Thus first graders devoted considerable resources to attending to words compared with other older readers. However, even adult readers had not achieved full automaticity. A second experiment produced similar results for identifying and classifying words, but without selective interference.

At the moment there is no compelling reason against arguing that logographic processing is a rudimentary form of lexical processing that becomes more automated for more frequent words. As readers gain more exposure to print their lexical processing of words becomes more developed in proportion to the extent of exposure. The net result is that after first grade there is a gradual speeding up in the process of word identification. It is still a matter of debate whether it can be argued that the change in speed after first grade is sharp enough to challenge the suggestion that essentially the same lexical process is taking place even in the first year or so of learning to read.

Could children with dyslexia who rely on logographic reading become fluent readers?

There is evidence that a proportion of children with dyslexia do become fluent readers, but in most cases we have no information whether they achieved this by relying mainly on logographic reading. An extreme example of achieving fluency is the case of a person with developmental dyslexia who eventually became a university professor (Rayner *et al.,* 1989). As we shall see briefly later, as an adult reader he had an ongoing visual problem which still made reading difficult.

Testing rather more subjects, Felton, Naylor and Wood (1990) studied 115 adults who had their reading well documented in childhood. Of these 115 subjects, 37 were reading disabled in childhood, 38 had been borderline and 40 had no reading difficulties. They showed that of the 37 who had been reading disabled in childhood, 19 (51%) were no longer in that category. These 19 subdivided into 10 who were borderline and 9 who had become average readers. When examining the borderline readers in childhood, 29 (76%) were reading fluently when they matured. Childhood and adult IQ scores were in the normal range for all groups.

Felton *et al.* also found that the phonetic decoding of nonwords and the manipulation of phonemes (tested by Felton *et al.* in adulthood) to be much worse for those adults classified as reading disabled in childhood compared with those who were not, even when controlling for intelligence and socioeconomic status. However, this difference could have been an effect of reading problems rather than a cause.

Nevertheless, it is instructive to see that many of the subjects deficient in sublexical processes in adulthood had had 'intense tutoring to teach sound-symbol associations and blending' (p. 494). Later we shall examine an experiment training sublexical skills in children with dyslexia which also concluded that such skills can be resistant to training (Lovett *et al.*, 1989). In the Felton *et al.* study it would have been interesting to examine those who were dyslexic as children to determine exactly what differentiated those who eventually learned to read from those who did not. For instance, to what extent do they still sustain their exposure to print? What, if any, is the difference in their nonword reading? This last point is relevant to a later discussion as it would reveal if some became fluent readers despite a dysfunctional/inoperable sublexical system.

It could be countered that in certain instances the reading of those previously classified as dyslexic may not be entirely normal. For instance, the undergraduate RE could not read new words without great difficulty; similarly, the university professor SJ, who had a visual reading problem, was taught to occlude his parafoveal field by a mechanical device in order to read 'normally'. Nevertheless, reading is no longer an impediment to their normal intellectual functioning. SJ, even before his 'treatment', had learned to cope with his affliction and do well at the professional level. In a few recorded cases, this has led to quite extraordinary levels of academic attainment.

Despite the suggestion that children with dyslexia could learn to read fluently by means of their lexical route, some have failed to become proficient. This could be because they have not had the appropriate learning conditions. Using an exclusive logographic route for normal reading is going to be a more disruptive activity when a new word or a vaguely familiar word is encountered. There will be no sublexical route to aid identification, so other methods have to be used. These methods will include simply asking someone (and in a good school or home environment, help may be readily available), using a dictionary that has pictorial and symbolic representations, or more recently, using a computer to access the spoken form of the word. Some form of analogy to other words stored lexically could be used. The child may also use the surrounding context of the word, but this can often be unsatisfactory and lead to a vaguer understanding of the passage of text. However, in normally developing readers context appears to be important when the word is on the borderline between familiarity and unfamiliarity (Adams and Huggins, 1985). We shall shortly examine one case study (JM) in which this was an obviously useful strategy.

One possible reason why there is such a high proportion of boys who are dyslexic is because having fewer social skills they find it more difficult to solicit help from others when stuck with words. However, boys enjoy using computers so the findings of studies such as Reitsma's (1988) could be useful. Reitsma displayed text on a computer screen with relatively difficult target words embedded in it. If the screen were touched at the location of the difficult word, the spoken word was given by the computer. This led to a significant improvement relative to children who passively read the text while listening to the spoken version. There have been several recent studies on the benefits of computers for training (e.g., van Daal and van der Leij, 1992).

In contrast to this social explanation of sex differences, Geschwind and Galaburda (1985a, b, c) have related the effects of testosterone on neural substrates, male gender differentiation, asymmetries in the structure of the brain and left handedness. They suggested that the asymmetries are connected with language learning difficulties especially in the case of dyslexia.

The discussion on long-term logographic development leads to a testable hypothesis which I shall put in strong terms as the 'logographic-to-fluency' hypothesis. The proposal is that children with dyslexia who are reading exclusively or predominantly by means of their lexical route will eventually become fluent readers if the following conditions are satisfied:

(1) that on close examination they have no potential visual processing problems, such as an interfering effect in the parafovea, or eye movement abnormalities, or pattern recognition deficiencies, particularly in feature discrimination. (See the chapters by Lovegrove and Stein in this volume for an elaboration.)

(2) that their listening comprehension is normal.

(3) that there are no signs of soft neurological impairment. These first three conditions would be satisfied because these fulfil some of the criteria of being dyslexic, previously mentioned.

(4) This is a very important element: that they have the means of identifying unfamiliar words close at hand whenever they are reading (e.g., by computer access).

(5) that they are given guidance and encouragement to keep selecting material for reading; and furthermore that stories are read to them to stimulate their interest in reading. The teacher might read passages that are too difficult. The main aspect about this particular element is that repeated exposure to print is a crucially important aspect of lexical development. Stanovich and West (1989) and West, Madison and Stanovich (1991) tested American adult readers in their reading competence and also gave them a test involving identifying authors from a list of authors' names from popular fiction and fake names. This test was used as an index of likely reading exposure. They found a good relationship between reading performance and identifying authors. Similar results have been found in children (Cunningham and Stanovich, 1991; Stanovich and Cunningham, 1992).

(6) that they are also encouraged to write about things that interest them on a regular (daily) basis. Writing, especially writing in which spelling is corrected, will help focus attention on the visual features of the words being read.

'Fluent reading' needs to be defined in this context as the ability to read passages of text with a speed and level of understanding commensurate with their age. But, if the text contains low-frequency words not previously encountered, they will still need to seek help in order to read them. RE is an example of such a person.

This hypothesis could be tested by means of an experiment that provided all the conditions outlined above. It could be called the 'fast word retrieval' experiment because the most essential component is to provide the appropriate word name as quickly as possible. The children would need to be checked that they were actually impoverished in their sublexical route. It may be that their sublexical development is poor but compatible with their reading age. An ethical decision would have to be taken whether training in sublexical processing would be denied them during the proposed experiment. This is a complex issue, but one way round it is to allow such training as long as it does not interfere with the main theme of fast word retrieval. If sublexical processing develops, this should be regarded as a bonus as it will mean that unfamiliar words can be decoded. But it masks the question whether exclusive lexical development can lead to fluent reading. Nevertheless, there are means of testing the operation of sublexical processes, so children who eventually achieve fluency without it will confirm the 'logographic-to-fluency' hypothesis.

If some children do not achieve fluency, even after several years, this would be confirmation of Nicolson and Fawcett's hypothesis that children with dyslexia have difficulty in achieving automaticity. But the argument might hinge on how long teachers (and learners) are willing to continue training to prove that they will not achieve automaticity. To a certain extent a motivational element is bound to be involved. For instance, in normally achieving readers there is a dip in reading for pleasure at about 13 years because of pressure of time from the school curriculum and from peers in evenings and at weekends. For readers who have dyslexia the situation is worse as they are trying to follow the curriculum impeded by their reading problems, so they have less time available for reading for pleasure if they are in a normal school environment.

The only concrete evidence for the hypothesis are cases such as RE who was seen at the end of the process, rather than during the time when she was learning to read. However, the following case study increases our understanding of reading development when there are problems with the sublexical route.

A longitudinal study of reading with minimal sublexical involvement

Snowling and Hulme (1989) reported a longitudinal study on a developmental phonological dyslexic (JM), who was tested between 8;5 years and 12;2 years. After initial testing JM was taught in a residential school and then a secondary school that taught by eclectic methods including teaching grapheme–phoneme correspondences. His WISC-R IQ was 123, he had phonological processing deficits including poor memory span. He did not appear to have visual processing abnormalities, giving a perfect reproduction of the Rey Osterrieth figure, which is a complex line drawing. More importantly, in the final session he was also very good at remembering sequences of letter-like abstract forms (2 standard deviations above the mean of reading age controls), which would imply that he would potentially not have problems with logographic processing.

His improvement in reading comprehension over this period was erratic but encouraging. He began at an age level of 6;8 (nearly two years behind), after 18 months it was 9;6, it stayed at the same level 12 months later, but rose to 11;1 years (only 13 months behind chronological age) one year later when he was 12 years old. On initial testing at 8;5 he was completely unable to read nonwords, while average performance of reading age-matched controls were 50% and 30% correct for reading aloud one- and two-syllable words, respectively. When tested four years later, these scores of the controls rose to 90% and 87%, respectively, but rose only to 26% and 25%, respectively, for JM. Thus at the age of 12 years, he was not entirely a phonological dyslexic as he was developing a primitive sublexical system. Snowling (personal communication, 1992) in fact would prefer to avoid the use of the term 'phonological dyslexia' because such cases all have primitive sublexical systems. These signs of a sublexical system are also supported by analysis of his reading errors and his performance in spelling. Further tests on being able to use context and on his reading comprehension produced good performance.

Snowling and Hulme conclude that JM finds it extremely difficult to improve on alphabetic skill despite four years of specialist remedial teaching. They attribute his slowness in acquiring sight vocabulary as due to, first, problems in output phonology, in particular he has voicing problems in his speech; and second, to poor knowledge of letters. One wonders if he had been given the 'fast word retrieval' environment described earlier, whether he would have acquired sight vocabulary at a quicker pace. What vocabulary he does have is as quickly retrieved on most occasions as normal controls (personal communication, 1992).

Snowling and Hulme regarded his ability to recognise words visually as 'very poor' (p. 399), presumably because on the Schonell Reading test his reading was over three years behind and because of the visual errors in his reading (e.g., *shin–skin, lever–level*). But his actual lexical development is probably masked by relying on this read-aloud test because of his problems of pronunciation.

It is interesting to note that his reading comprehension was only one year behind. This at least indicates that his comprehension ability is good. Difficult words on the Neale reading test are spoken for the child. Thus reading difficulty on the comprehension reading test only serves to slow down the rate of 'reading'. His heavy dependence on contextual and semantic information seems to be sustaining his reading development, so that his reading comprehension is only one year behind.

The latest study of JM (Hulme and Snowling, 1992), tested at the age of 13, shows essentially the same characteristics as before, except that they omitted his comprehension reading age. This time they examined his nonword reading in detail and showed a lack of phonology in reading but a sensitivity to the visual similarity of the nonwords to real words.

To conclude so far, it is proposed that children with dyslexia with severe problems in sublexical processes could learn to become fluent, automatic readers providing a number of qualifying conditions are satisfied, particularly the element called 'fast word retrieval', which enables reading to continue without too much disruption. The evidence suggests that for some individuals with impaired phonology it can be extremely difficult, if not impossible, to learn to use a sublexical route involving grapheme–phoneme conversion. But at the moment there is only converging evidence from disparate sources to support these conclusions rather than actual confirmatory evidence. We shall return to this issue in the final section.

DEVELOPMENT OF SUBLEXICAL SKILLS

It is clear from the previous discussion that development of logographic skills without the assistance of sublexical processing is slower, sometimes much slower, than normal. We also saw how for some readers with phonological difficulties acquisition of a sublexical route is painfully slow, sometimes impossible, despite intensive coaching. John Rack's chapter (this volume) already covers phonological skills and I have dealt with the development of sublexical processes in detail elsewhere (e.g., Beech, 1989), so the following section on the normally achieving reader will be briefer than the volume of literature perhaps warrants.

So far the view has been taken that even children without sublexical skills, particularly in letter-sound decoding and sound blending, should become fluent readers as long as certain conditions are satisfied. Nevertheless, this does not imply that sublexical skills are unimportant, it simply implies that they may not be a necessary condition for fluent reading.

There is now a reasonable body of knowledge on the development of sublexical skills in the normally achieving reader and how these facilitate reading. We shall briefly examine a selection of this evidence and then turn to the evidence from dyslexic readers, which unfortunately is rather more sparse.

Development of reading and phonology in normally achieving readers

One demonstration of the importance of sublexical knowledge comes from examining the relationship between prior knowledge of letter sounds and phonological skills and the relationship between these skills and subsequent reading. Stuart and Coltheart (1988), mentioned earlier, demonstrated that prior phonological and letter-sound knowledge were significant predictors of reading age, even after the first year at school. Similarly, Lundberg, Olofsson and Wall (1980) found that reading and spelling in school could be predicted from prior skills in phonemic awareness some time before the beginning of formal reading training. Such findings challenge the stage view of Frith, that the first stage of reading is purely logographic if phonological processes can be implicated in early reading development.

Wagner and Torgesen (1987) distinguished 'phonological recoding in lexical access' from 'phonological awareness'. The former means that characters are decoded into sounds in order to access their lexical referent. Awareness of phonology refers to an explicit knowledge of the sounds in words. Wagner and Torgesen reanalysed the data from the Lundberg *et al.* study and other such studies and found a causal role for phonological awareness. However, necessary information on prior and concurrent knowledge of logographic skills was missing from this analysis (which Wagner and Torgesen acknowledge) as it is possible for such developing reading skills to influence phonological awareness.

Bradley and Bryant (1983), in a seminal experiment, showed that training letter-sound knowledge helped reading development, while training in phonemic awareness just failed to improve reading significantly. However this lack of effect for phonemic awareness training was not found by Lundberg, Frost and Petersen (1988) who intensively trained a large number of children for 8 months in the absence of a reading programme. Reading performance subsequently improved relative to controls, but as the children were Swedish the orthographic regularity of their language would make such training more worthwhile than for English children.

Wagner (1988) performed a meta-analysis on a total of 16 longitudinal and training studies. Among the criteria for inclusion for the longitudinal analysis was that an initial test was undertaken at kindergarten when reading was at best rudimentary. Estimates of *rho* were made, which is a measure of the population correlation between two variables. With a couple of exceptions, the magnitude of the estimates of the causal relations between phonological processing (based on phonemes and syllables) and reading skill was substantial for the longitudinal studies. (This is *not* due to the phenomenon of obtaining significance because of large subject numbers.) However, the estimates based on the training studies were doubled. Several interesting aspects emerge from this meta-analysis:

(1) IQ was probably not a moderator variable as partialling it out did not affect a subsequent path analysis. This could imply that differences in intelligence will not impede the likelihood of subsequent success in phonemic training.

(2) It demonstrates the importance of training skills in phonological processing in order to prevent subsequent reading problems.

(3) Each of four phonological processing abilities had a causal influence on word analysis skills. These skills were the analysis and synthesis of phonemes, coding in the context of lexical

analysis and coding in working memory. Taking these in turn, analysis involved segmenting words into units, usually phonemes or syllables. Synthesis, often referred to as 'blending', required combining segments of a word into a whole word. These first two skills tap important skills for grapheme–phoneme translation. Analysis would be important for the process of breaking letters into appropriate segments and generating their sounds. However, initial division of letters into their constituent graphemes (e.g., *shout* has three graphemes to convert to phonemes) would be an important additional skill not tested here. Synthesis, which was the most important of the skills, would be useful for then blending these phonemes together to produce candidate phonological strings.

The third skill with a causal role was coding/lexical access, referring to the accessing of a word's meaning from its phonological code. Thus after blending, this kind of lexical access would be the final stage. The fourth skill, coding in working memory, enables phonemes to be retained in memory while the operation involving their blending is sustained. Perhaps the order that Wagner ascribed the third and fourth skills ought to have been reversed in terms of their probable order of operation during execution.

A second path analysis on word recognition skill produced similar results, except that synthesis produced a negative but significant path coefficient indicating that it was suppressing some variance of the other skills.

(4) The fourth finding of note in Wagner's analysis was that word analysis skills had a causal role in the development of the skills of analysis and in coding in working memory, but not on synthesis skills. Due to paucity of data, only word analysis out of the two reading skills was examined and one of the four phonological processing skills was omitted (recoding/lexical access).

These results concur with the proposition of Perfetti *et al.* (1987) that the skill of synthesis in particular is an aid to subsequent reading, while the process of learning to read facilitates the development of word analysis. The findings also support a componential approach to reading skills (e.g., Beech, 1989; Schwartz, 1984) suggesting that reading skill itself consists of a number of component skills. One major thrust of research into reading has been to determine the nature of these skills and their relative roles in reading development. The set of skills related to sublexical development appears to be trainable for the majority of children and to have an important impact on subsequent reading development. Just how the sublexical processes might interact with lexical development will be discussed later.

An element missing from the training studies reviewed by Wagner is that there is no explicit part in the programmes for explaining to the children how such skills should be deployed. Cunningham (1990) compared a 'skill and drill' training method to teach phonemic awareness and letter-sound coding with one involving the children being explicitly taught the value of such skills. She showed that adding the metalinguistic aspect improved performance in reading.

Unfortunately, it is difficult to know whether metalinguistic awareness was actually excluded from training by individual trainers in the reviewed studies. It would be tempting for teachers, having trained a phonological skill, to attempt to show how this skill would be used, and thus impart metalinguistic awareness. Clarification of the matter would mean measuring the level of skill development, and the extent of its transferability within the appropriate context. If there has been a change in the way that (say) unfamiliar words are tackled, this would be an indication of success. This could be backed up by detailed questioning of the children to see if they can throw any light on the matter.

The unit of analysis in the sublexical route

The debate about the unit of analysis in sublexical coding (apart from the debate of whether sublexical coding even exists e.g., Humphreys and Evett, 1985) is focused on the situation where the child encounters an unfamiliar word. Experimentalists have presented nonwords to developing readers to simulate this situation to examine how well they cope. As Coltheart *et al.* (1983) explain, the orthographic unit could be the grapheme (already described) and the phonological unit the phoneme. Correspondences are learned between the two. Second, correspondences could be formed between strings of one or more graphemes and phonemes. Third, the system could be morphemic so that there are correspondences between morphemes and phonological codes. Finally, the activation of an orthographic string activates neighbours of words with similar orthographic strings. Since the time that paper was written (and before it), several different permutations of these possibilities have been proposed (e.g., Patterson and Morton, 1985).

Coltheart *et al.* argued that it can be demonstrated experimentally whether a reader can parse graphemes during reading, because nonwords such as *zwuk* can only be read in this way. Such nonwords contain no morphemes, orthographic neighbours or consecutive letters that appear in any English words. But they conceded that such correspondences could be part of a broader system of orthographic–phonological correspondences. Could they have foreseen that connectionism was on the horizon?

Could any alternative from grapheme-to-phoneme conversion still be considered as a sublexical route, and what is the important distinguishing features between the two? In this connectionist era it is becoming increasingly difficult to define neat boxes that contain certain processes, although the practice is still prevalent in cognitive neuropsychology. For example, we have the strange situation of a lexical route being simulated by a connectionist model (as already described) that does not actually have lexical representations. The basic distinction between lexicon and sublexical processes could be that in fluent reading on the one hand, familiar words are identified rapidly by a lexical process; but less familiar words, on the other, are decoded by a more complicated process which is open to several possibilities.

The connectionist version would be that less frequent exposures lead to slower responses, but the process is still basically the same as for identifying familiar words. Thus decoding such words does not involve a sublexical process. On the other hand, a sublexical process invokes some other kind of alternative analysis, involving in many cases a phonological process, which leads to lexical access.

There are further problems such as whether these proceed in parallel, whether a race takes place between the alternative systems, whether the sublexical process operates exclusively, and so on. Thus in answer to the question, other forms apart from grapheme conversion would still be considered as sublexical. The exception is when all phenomena are explained in terms of the characteristic of one route. The parsimonious connectionist model of Seidenberg and McClelland has proved seductive, but it does have its detractors (e.g., Besner *et al.* , 1990).

There has been much recent work on the role of subsyllabic units of analysis and their role in reading (e.g., see Goswami and Bryant, 1990). For example, Treiman, Goswami and Bruck (1990) compared the reading of two types of consonant-vowel-consonant (CVC) nonwords. The real word neighbours of one type shared their VC units, while the other sort shared with few or no real words. They found that all categories of reader that they tested from first grade to adult were better at reading those nonwords with common VC units. This was in contrast to reading the initial CV units. One implication of such work is that the use of nonword reading as a means of measuring sublexical involvement has to be interpreted cautiously. The fact that word neighbourhoods are influencing nonword reading demonstrates that the application of grapheme–phoneme correspondence rules is not the only process that may be operating.

Closer examination of their results revealed that lexicalisation errors were more prevalent in nonwords with neighbours and this became more important as reading skill developed. Nevertheless, children even at the end of first grade were affected by neighbourhood effects. Goswami and Bryant (1990) suggest that because of early experiences with rhyme, readers make use of onset and rime units at the beginning of learning to read. Treiman *et al.* come to the sensible conclusion that there are relative merits for both grapheme–phoneme conversion models and analogy-based models (see Patterson and Coltheart, 1987), which is why reference is made in this chapter to 'sublexical' processes.

The role of sublexical skills in dyslexia

We have seen how component skills within sublexical processes have significant causal roles in the development of analytical reading (Wagner, 1988). Such training might also be suitable for helping those with dyslexia overcome their disabilities. Reviews of the treatment literature were generally pessimistic in the early 1980s about which were the most effective treatments for dyslexia (Gittleman, 1983; Hewison, 1982; Johnson, 1978). The view that has been taken earlier here is that the training of sublexical skills for children with dyslexia can be very difficult in some cases. For instance, RE had problems in phonological memory which could have incapacitated the efficient operation of grapheme–phoneme conversion, and similarly, JM had problems with output phonology which could have affected sublexical developments. It is possible that certain subskills necessary for efficient sublexical operations are not supported by the necessary underlying cognitive systems for certain children presenting dyslexic symptoms. This is not to imply that this underlying problem is connected to brain morphology. Current evidence for the neurological basis of dyslexia is actually quite weak, particularly because of the lack of appropriate controls (Hynd and Semrud-Clikeman, 1989).

Since the doldrums of the early 1980s an impressively ambitious treatment programme for children with dyslexia has been undertaken by Lovett *et al.* (1989) which breaks new ground from previous research and is worth close scrutiny. They randomly allocated 178 children into one of three treatments: a 'decoding skills' group who were trained in word recognition and spelling, an 'oral and written language development' group, and a treatment control group who were allocated the same amount of time and attention, but were taught about classroom survival skills. Thus they controlled for the 'Hawthorne' effect by making comparison with a control group that was treated similarly in every respect apart from being given the direct treatment.

The 'decoding skills' (DS) group were trained predominantly in word recognition, but there was an accompanying element of training sublexical skills. In fact, their aim for this group was that they should acquire rapid word recognition appropriate for their age level. For instance, Lovett (1987) is cited as demonstrating that subgroups of the sample when compared to age- and IQ-matched normal readers were inferior in word recognition in terms of accuracy, speed or both. They also aimed to improve spelling. The programme involved a very large corpus of words. The regular words were introduced in families (e.g., fade, jade, made). These were trained to a different method than for irregular words. Regular words had their letter-sound correspondences emphasised, whereas the irregular words were taught by sight methods alone. Difficulty was graded by frequency for the irregular words and by letter-sound correspondence difficulty for the regular words. They also trained previously mentioned skills: phonetic analysis and blending. In addition they trained rapid word recognition, morphological analysis and spelling. Note that everything was restricted to the domain of single word-in-isolation reading or spelling.

The second group had the 'Oral and Written Language Simulation' (OWLS) programme. This was prompted by proposals (e.g., Denckla, 1979) that children with problems of dyslexia also have speech and language development problems. The lower language skills covered included phonological processing and rapid print-to-sound naming, so there was some overlap with the first group. But the principal aim was to train semantic and linguistic facets of analysis.

Each of the three groups had 40 sessions altogether of 50-60 minutes' duration, four times a week for 10 weeks. Training was sampled by observers naive to group membership and the purpose of the study. The children were aged between 8 and 13 years. Although selected because of a specific reading difficulty, and selected on the basis of the usual exclusionary criteria and labelled as 'dyslexic' in the title of the paper, the authors do not appear to have included home background as one of their criteria of exclusion. Socioeconomic data were only available on a third of the sample and 71% of these were in the middle ranges. Thus it is probable that a small proportion of the children were poor readers because of an environmental factor. Nevertheless, they did attend the clinic, which suggests an element of parental motivation. Most of the readers (60%) had problems in decoding accuracy (at least 1.5 years below expectation). The rest were disabled in terms of reading rate (at least 1.5 years below expectation), but close to accuracy expectations. Those with selective comprehension problems were excluded.

They presented a battery of different tests prior to and after training and found that some of the subskill problems associated with dyslexia could be remediated, so that, for example, the DS group made 'sizeable word recognition gains' (p. 110), but their knowledge of grapheme–phoneme correspondence skills did not improve. Thus they failed to improve in reading nonwords, indicating that the improvement in word recognition skills was not gained by an improvement in grapheme–phoneme correspondence skills. This supports the earlier contention that in some cases it would be better to concentrate on improving lexical rather than sublexical processes. This group also improved more with the exception words compared with the regular words. This intriguing result is likely to be due to more time being allowed for individual exception words. The regular words were introduced in families so that individual time for specific words was reduced. The frequency of exposure principle has already been advocated as perhaps the most important determinant of lexical reading performance.

Overall the two experimental groups improved relative to the controls in word recognition and some measures of spelling performance. Specific improvements for the OWLS group were observed on measures related to the training; however, these skills did not appear to transfer to other tests purporting to measure the same skills. Nevertheless, they improved in reading accuracy, rate and comprehension, vocabulary and in aspects of semantic and syntactic skills. For both groups (DS and OWLS), the 40 hours of training did not appear to affect contextual reading of other tests or spelling knowledge needed for real words.

There were some isolated gains in phonological processes, so that the DS group improved only in sound blending. Both the DS and OWLS groups improved in letter-naming speed. Thus certain component skills for sublexical processing could be capable of training. One has also got to bear in mind the limited time period. It is possible that with an accompanying instruction in metalinguistic awareness and more training time many of these children could have been encouraged to tackle unfamiliar words using sublexical processes. On the other hand, it may be better to devote most resources to the lexical route, considering that this seems to be the one that most responds to training in those readers suffering from dyslexia.

One possibility for teachers would be to undertake a similar training programme. If there is an improvement in word recognition over the training period, then teaching resources could be concentrated on this. There would be no harm in including training programmes to improve comprehension as well, even though the evidence from this particular study suggests a problem of domain-specificity. For instance, remember that JM's reading comprehension was considerably ahead of his apparent word recognition skills. His skills in comprehension appeared to be compensating for sublexical deficit.

Conners and Olson's work (1990) on children with dyslexia also suggests reliance on comprehension skills. When matched to a younger group of normally achieving readers on word recognition, their listening and reading comprehension was found to be significantly higher, but sublexical processing was significantly worse.

These results of Lovett *et al.* also concur with Snowling's on a smaller scale (1980; 1981) that a group of children with dyslexia improved in reading with age due to improvements in sight vocabulary rather than by improving in the use of grapheme–phoneme correspondence rules. The great difficulty in training these correspondence rules could link in with the finding of a hereditary connection with phonological coding, whereas there is an environmental connection with word recognition skills (Olson *et al.*, 1989).

However, the results of a training study persuade Olson *et al.* to have a different view concerning the ease of training the sublexical skills of children with dyslexia. They had reading disabled subjects undergo an average of about 10 hours of training by computer. The subjects were described as 'disabled readers' and as having specific reading difficulty. But as 51 were taken from only three different American schools (in contrast to Lovett *et al.*'s sample), one wonders if the children were actually poor readers, rather than children with dyslexia. Four groups read stories on the screen and obtained speech feedback (by targeting unknown words), which was the whole word, the syllables, the subsyllables or a combination. They had regular tests of comprehension which indicated that they were comprehending the materials well. The training programme appears to be excellent as it combines the reading of (presumably) interesting material with learning painlessly about lexical and sublexical processes.

Olson *et al.* had a control group, but as it was not given the equivalent training attention, we shall ignore it for our purposes. They suffered from a shortage of subjects, with numbers at the end of training varying from 6 to 10. There were modest gains in word recognition for all four groups (15%, 7%, 14% and 13%, respectively) in recognising words targeted on the screen. There was also evidence that many new words were being learned during the experiment which had not been targeted, and which presumably learned outside the programme. Most important from our perspective was their finding that experiencing segmented feedback helped nonword reading significantly better than whole-word reading. But neither the magnitude of the effect nor the significance level are reported. Conners and Olson (1990) referring to this work state: 'recent research with computer-based reading and speech feedback for decoding difficulties has shown substantial gains for dyslexic readers' phonological coding and word recognition'.

The apparent contradiction between the findings of the Lovett *et al.* work and Olson *et al.* could be due to the nature of the subjects used in the two studies or to the type of training programmes that were used. As the old cliché goes: further research is required.

Resistance to developing lexical skills

Having suggested that a proportion of children with dyslexia might benefit from direct word recognition training, it is salutary to consider a relatively small number of readers who either choose not to use this skill, but can do so, or who *may* be unable to use this skill. Such readers have been described as letter-by-letter readers and as surface dyslexics. These are usually regarded as two distinct categories.

Surface dyslexics are supposed to be characterised by irregularly spelled words being read incorrectly (e.g., *tread* read as *treed*) as if grapheme–phoneme correspondence rules had been applied. Another aspect is that homographs that differentiate meanings by spelling pattern are not distinguished. Spelling is impaired as most errors tend to be phonologically correct.

A developmental dyslexic (referred to as CD) with these characteristics was studied by Coltheart *et al.* (1983). She was tested between the ages of 15 and $16\frac{1}{2}$ years and had a delay in reading of between 4 to 6 years, with her spelling lagging even further behind. However, her reading performance for irregular words compared with regular was 90% to 67% correct (both out of 39), which is not a large difference, especially when there are no reading age controls for comparison. It was later shown that normally progressing younger readers matched to the level of CD also had problems with irregular words (Bryant and Impey, 1986). Furthermore, Wilding (1989) pointed out several aspects to question the diagnosis of Coltheart *et al.*: her nonword reading was very poor at 31%, suggesting problems in sublexical processing; and there was insufficient evidence from the data given to justify their claims of her predominantly using regularisation in pronunciation. The evidence instead suggested a mixture of impoverished lexical access and the application of sublexical processes, but there was not enough information to be sure.

There actually seems to be a paucity of evidence for the so-called surface dyslexia syndrome. For example, Wilding (1989) went on to reanalyse the reading errors of the surface dyslexics studied by Holmes (1973) and again showed poor nonword reading coupled with evidence of visual errors in reading.

Hanley, Hastie and Kay (1992) suggest that the low incidence is because such surface dyslexics can get by with using their sublexical processes to read regular words and use their logographic strategies for the more frequently encountered irregular words. This means that they will be able to cover up much of their reading difficulties. But according to Frith (1985) surface dyslexics will encounter problems in spelling because the room for error is greater when translating phonemes to graphemes. Hanley *et al.* present the case of a man in his early twenties, called Allan, whose oral reading is prompt and whose nonword reading and spelling is accurate; however he has a spelling age of about 9 years.

They demonstrated that he had neither phonological problems nor visual problems and that the vast majority of his spelling errors were phonological in nature. Despite the claims of Coltheart *et al.* that surface dyslexics should have differences between reading regular and irregular words, there seems to be no noticeable difference in Allan; but this could have been due to a ceiling effect. As his reading was apparently fluent, reaction time measures should have been tried. The evidence that his reading was different from normal came from a lexical decision task in which the letter strings failed to match in the beginning, middle or end of the word. Normal performance for the 'different' responses is for the middle part to be slower than the end positions, but Allan demonstrated fast left-to-right scanning of the letter strings. In addition there was a word superiority effect of 156 ms, similar to a control subject. But the word superiority effect for the 'different' responses failed to reach significance. Examination of the magnitude of the reaction times suggests that all strings were scanned left to right and if a match occurred the search terminated. Thus positive responses appear from my inspection to be the same as if all characters had been scanned. But his word superiority effect does not show that his rate of scanning the letters of words was faster; rather, that an effect was occurring on the whole word. An unusual aspect was that the visual angle of presentation was quite wide for the longest strings, which may have exaggerated scanning times. Letter length was manipulated, but no statistics are reported on whether this was influential; presumably it was not.

The picture that seems to emerge is that he reads words swiftly from left to right, but both lexical and sublexical processes are in operation because he commits both visual reading errors and regularises irregular words. Furthermore he demonstrates a word superiority effect. He appears to have no problems making auditory judgements concerning rhymes, a task that we saw earlier RE had problems with. He appears to have found it difficult to learn to read and at present he does not read for pleasure. In this respect his reading may be fast, but it appears to be dysfunctional. Some possibilities are that he has an abnormally slow grapheme–phoneme correspondence system (relative to fluent readers) that (1) confirms prior lexical analysis or (2) generates phonological strings for lexical analysis or (3) both lexical and sublexical systems race against each other.

An interesting question to pose, especially from a remediation viewpoint, is why did Allan develop this way? Goulandris and Snowling (1991) report a similar case except that she had a poor visual memory which could explain her syndrome. But in Allan's case there is no test that has been reported that would explain why he has had problems with logographic/lexical processing. Therefore, it seems that further testing/remediation is necessary to establish whether Allan is an *elective* surface dyslexic. This is assuming that the label 'surface dyslexic' is used as a shorthand term which does not preclude the possibility of some degree of lexical involvement.

One direction would be to tackle his problems in spelling. As we saw in the Lovett *et al.* study it is possible to train spelling in children with dyslexia. For a limited period of time Allan could have a programme of remediation in the spelling of a small set of irregular words. If he is able to improve, perhaps at a rate comparable to spelling dyslexic controls, this would suggest that his problems in spelling have arisen due to inappropriate strategies. If that works, and if Allan is sufficiently motivated, a similar programme might be attempted for reading, perhaps by devising a programme that encourages an increased exposure to print by reading for pleasure.

Hanley *et al.* end by commenting that it is important to find children who are developing skills similar to Allan to monitor their phonological skills. It was only when Allan was 12 years old that he was given special help and even then it was only in the form of special English classes and concessionary marking. If such reading and spelling problems had been tackled earlier, it may have been easier to remedy them.

THE INTERACTION BETWEEN LEXICAL AND SUBLEXICAL PROCESSES

According to evidence already reviewed, the development of a sublexical route in normally achieving readers aids reading development, and reading in turn helps phonemic awareness. However, children with dyslexia who are trained in lexical and sublexical reading skills appear to improve in word recognition skills but (within the period of a training programme) do not improve in sublexical processes (although it should be added that evidence from Olson *et al.*, 1990, on a small set of reading disabled subjects might suggest otherwise). Furthermore, there is evidence to suggest that problems in grapheme–phoneme processing in the reading disabled is genetically determined, whereas lexical development is more environmentally determined.

One might take at least two theoretical perspectives on this evidence, as starkly outlined above. One is the Matthew effect theory (Stanovich, 1986) and the other is that sublexical route development for some reading disabled children is too difficult to be viable, to be called the Intractable Sublexical Development (ISD) hypothesis.

The Matthew effect argues that the better readers get better and the poor readers get poorer, relative to each other. This is not a hypothesis at this point, it is simply a description of the data. This effect is predicted, according to Stanovich, if there is a reciprocal causal relationship, which appears to be the case for reading performance and the development of sublexical processes. This means that poor readers have less exposure to print because of their poor phonological abilities. Conversely, those with good grapheme–phoneme and other related skills can sustain their reading. They encounter more print and their logographic/lexical system develops at a faster rate. The previously reviewed meta-analysis by Wagner (1988) lends support for this interpretation in demonstrating that four distinct phonological skills determine reading and certain of these skills are determined by reading. However, there are still gaps in the evidence concerning the precise nature of the influence of reading on phonological development.

The ISD hypothesis proposes that success in the training of sublexical skills is likely in most cases, but there will be a hard core of children who are lacking in a prerequisite phonological skill necessary for successful development of certain types of sublexical skills, particularly those involving grapheme–phoneme conversion. Such cases are currently termed phonological dyslexics. For example, RE, who was a fluent reader, had a deficient phonological memory as indicated by a poor memory for digit span.

The main contrast between the Matthew effect and the ISD hypothesis is that the Matthew effect predicts the likelihood that training will induce all dyslexic readers to use a sublexical route to decode unfamiliar words and that this in turn would help their reading development. However, I do not think that Stanovich would intend such a strong interpretation as there could be other factors that could account for failure, such as lack of motivation.

The ISD hypothesis has the following implication for remediation. A sustained programme of training should be given to the dyslexic reader on sublexical processing, word recognition and training on how to use sublexical processes for unfamiliar words. Exactly the same programme should be given to younger children of the same reading age. The programme should monitor progress in the use of grapheme–phoneme skills and related skills as well as word recognition development. At the end of the programme if the dyslexic child is failing to make any progress in sublexical processes relative to the controls, remediation should then concentrate on developing word exposure as outlined earlier. This is not to say that sublexical training should be completely discontinued or not brought back at a later point. The decision to discontinue (or de-emphasise) sublexical training should be taken in conjunction with evidence that suggests that one or more component skills of sublexical development are seriously dysfunctional.

One criticism of the ISD hypothesis might be that it appears to be making a distinction between readers who are dyslexic and normally achieving readers matched to them in reading age, by suggesting that some children with dyslexia would not benefit from sublexical training. Some would suggest that children with dyslexia in relation to reading age controls are very similar to one another. For instance, Beech and Harding (1984) motivated by a developmental lag hypothesis demonstrated a lack of difference between poor readers and such controls in phonological and sublexical processes and this was followed up and replicated by Treiman and Hirsh-Pasek (1985), Bruck (1989) and others, this time on children with dyslexia.

But the outcome of this debate is by no means conclusive, as the review by Olson *et al.* (1990) shows, there are considerable differences between studies. One prediction of the ISD hypothesis would be that older children with dyslexia would be more likely to be different from reading age controls, because their phonological skills would remain relatively undeveloped in relation to word recognition skills. Such lexical skills would be developing as a function of frequency of exposure. There is some support for this position from the studies reviewed by Olson *et al.* In addition, a study by Johnston, Rugg and Scott (1987) making a direct age comparison found a lack of deficit in nonword reading for 8-year-old poor readers, but a difference for 11-year-olds.

Olson *et al.* in their review also suggested that when the samples were dyslexic readers, significant deficiencies in phonological coding were manifest relative to poor readers. But recently, Beech and Awaida (1992) studied nonword reading in depth in 9-year-old poor readers and found problems relative to normally achieving reading controls matched both in reading and phonemic processing. This result indicated that problems in sublexical processing may not be confined to readers with dyslexia and that they can occur for poor readers with a reading age as young as 9 years. Care was taken in this study to eliminate possible priming effects which may have masked potential nonword reading deficiencies in previous work.

The ISD hypothesis would apply to a proportion, probably a small proportion, of children with dyslexia. This implies that although children with dyslexia have been discussed collectively, the previously predicted outcomes (e.g., intractability in training grapheme–phoneme conversion) are more likely for some, while others may show a tendency in the predicted direction.

Designations such as 'surface dyslexia' and 'phonological dyslexia' can lead to over-simplified conceptions of reading development which may lead to a misguided assumption of a reciprocity in the predominant use of lexical or sublexical processes. Wilding (1989) in particular is critical of making such exclusive categorisations, preferring to note that all the cases he reviewed simply involved deficits in phonological processes. But at the time he would have been unaware of the case of JAS (Goulandris and Snowling, 1991) who seems to have normal phonological processing in reading, but has problems in visual memory. Consequently JAS appears to have difficulties in feature analysis when reading.

What has been argued for here is the feasibility of distinguishing between tractable strategic problems in lexical and sublexical skills and those that are intractable. There are means to investigate these that can have important consequences on future remediation. It has been suggested that as long as there are no apparent visual memory impairments, readers should be encouraged to develop reading using lexical processes. But there is also strong evidence for the reciprocal nature of phonological and reading processes so that most developing readers would benefit from sublexical training (and training inducing metalinguistic awareness); but in the few cases of severe deficit in phonology, it may be better to put less emphasis on sublexical training and concentrate on other strengths.

ACKNOWLEDGEMENT

The author is grateful to Professor Margaret Snowling for comments on an earlier version of this chapter.

REFERENCES

Adams, M.J. and Huggins, A.W.F. (1985). The growth of children's sight vocabulary: A quick test with educational and theoretical implications. *Reading Research Quarterly, 20*, 262–281.

Beech, J. R. (1989). The componential approach to learning reading skills. In A. M. Colley and J. R. Beech (Eds.), *The Acquisition and Performance of*

Cognitive Skills (pp. 187–211). Chichester: Wiley.

Beech, J.R. and Awaida, M. (1992). Lexical and nonlexical routes: A comparison between normally achieving and poor readers. *Journal of Learning Disabilities*, *25*, 196–206.

Beech, J.R. and Harding, L. (1984). Phonemic processing and the poor reader from a developmental lag viewpoint. *Reading Research Quarterly*, *19*, 357–366.

Beech, J.R. and Harris, M. (1994). The prelingually deaf young reader: A case of logographic reading? Paper submitted for publication.

Besner, D., Twilley, L., McCann, R.S. and Seergobin, K. (1990). On the connection between connectionism and data: Are a few words necessary? *Psychological Review*, *97*, 432–46.

Bradley, L. and Bryant, P.E. (1983). Categorizing sounds and learning to read: A causal connection. *Nature*, *301*, 419–421.

Bruck, M. (1989). The word recognition and spelling of dyslexic children. *Reading Research Quarterly*, *24*, 51–69.

Bryant, P.E. and Impey, L. (1986). The similarities between normal readers and developmental and acquired dyslexics. *Cognition*, *24*, 121–137.

Campbell, R. and Butterworth, B. (1985). Phonological dyslexia and dysgraphia in a highly literate subject: A developmental case and associated deficits of phonemic processing and awareness. *Quarterly Journal of Experimental Psychology*, *37A*, 435–475.

Coltheart, M. (1978). Lexical access in simple reading tasks. In G. Underwood (Ed.), *Strategies of Information Processing* (pp. 151–216). London: Academic Press.

Coltheart, M., Masterson, J., Byng, S., Prior, M. and Riddoch, J. (1983). Surface dyslexia. *Quarterly Journal of Experimental Psychology*, *35A*, 469–495.

Conners, F.A. and Olson, R.K. (1990). Reading comprehension and normal readers: A component–skills analysis. In D.A. Balota, G.B. Flores d'Arcais and K. Rayner (Eds.), *Comprehension Processes in Reading*. Hillsdale, NJ: Erlbaum.

Cunningham, A.E. (1990). Explicit versus implicit instruction in phonemic awareness. *Journal of Experimental Child Psychology*, *50*, 429–444.

Cunningham, A.E. and Stanovich, K.E. (1991). Tracking the unique effects of print exposure in children: Associations with vocabulary, general knowledge and spelling. *Journal of Educational Psychology*, *83*, 264–274.

Denckla, M.B. (1979). Childhood learning disabilities. In K.M. Heilman and E. Valenstein (Eds.), *Clinical Neuropsychology*. New York: Oxford University Press.

Felton, R.H., Naylor, C.E. and Wood, F.B. (1990). Neuropsychological profile of adult dyslexics. *Brain and Language*, *39*, 485–497.

Frith, U. (1985). Beneath the surface of developmental dyslexia. In K.E.

Patterson, J.C. Marshall and M. Coltheart (Eds.), *Surface Dyslexia*. London: Routledge and Kegan Paul.

Gaines, R., Mandler, J.M. and Bryant, P. (1981). Immediate and delayed recall by hearing and deaf children. *Journal of Speech and Hearing Research, 24,* 463–469.

Geschwind, N. and Galaburda, A.M. (1985a). Cerebral lateralization: Biological mechanisms, associations, and pathology: I. A hypothesis and a program for research. *Archives of Neurology, 42,* 428–459.

Geschwind, N. and Galaburda, A.M. (1985b). Cerebral lateralization: Biological mechanisms, associations, and pathology: II. A hypothesis and a program for research. *Archives of Neurology, 42,* 521–552.

Geschwind, N. and Galaburda, A.M. (1985c). Cerebral lateralization: Biological mechanisms, associations, and pathology: III. A hypothesis and a program for research. *Archives of Neurology, 42,* 634–654.

Gittleman, R. (1983). Treatment of reading disorders. In M. Rutter (Ed.), *Developmental Neuropsychiatry.* New York: Guilford Press.

Goswami, U. and Bryant, P. (1990). *Phonological Skill and Learning to Read.* Hove: Erlbaum.

Goulandris, N.K. and Snowling, M.J. (1991). Visual memory deficits: A plausible cause of developmental dyslexia: Evidence from a single case study. *Cognitive Neuropsychology, 8,* 127–154.

Hanley, J.R., Hastie, K. and Kay, J. (1992). Developmental surface dyslexia and dysgraphia: an orthographic processing impairment. *Quarterly Journal of Experimental Psychology, 44A,* 285–319.

Harris, M. and Coltheart, M. (1986). *Language Processing in Children and Adults.* London: Routledge.

Hewison, J. (1982). The current status of remedial intervention for children with reading problems. *Developmental Medicine and Child Neurology, 24,* 183–186.

Holmes, J.M. (1973). *Dyslexia: A neurolinguistic study of traumatic and developmental disorders of reading.* Unpublished PhD thesis, University of Edinburgh.

Horn, C.C. and Manis, F.R. (1987). Development of automatic and speeded reading of printed words. *Journal of Experimental Child Psychology, 44,* 92–108.

Hulme, C. and Snowling, M. (1992). Deficits in output phonology: An explanation of reading failure? *Cognitive Neuropsychology, 9,* 47–72.

Humphreys, G.W. and Evett, L.J. (1985). Are there independent lexical and non–lexical routes in word processing? An evaluation of the dual–route theory of reading. *Behavioral and Brain Sciences, 8,* 689–740.

Hynd, G.W. and Semrud–Clikeman, M. (1989). Dyslexia and brain morphology. *Psychological Bulletin, 106,* 447–482.

Johnson, D.J. (1978). Remedial approaches to dyslexia. In A.L. Benton and D.

Pearl (Eds.), *Dyslexia: An appraisal of current knowledge*. New York: Oxford University Press.

Johnston, R.J., Rugg, M.D. and Scott, T. (1987). The influence of phonology on good and poor readers when reading for meaning. *Journal of Memory and Language, 26,* 57–68.

Kimura, Y. and Bryant, P.E. (1983). Reading and writing in English and Japanese: A cross–sectional study of young children. *British Journal of Developmental Psychology, 1,* 143–154.

Lovett, M.W. (1987). A developmental approach to reading disability: Accuracy and speed criteria of normal and deficient reading skill. *Child Development, 58,* 234–260.

Lovett, M.W., Ransby, M.J., Hardwick, N., Johns, M.S. and Donaldson, S.A. (1989). Can dyslexia be treated? Treatment–specific and generalized effects in dyslexic children's response to remediation. *Brain and Language, 37,* 90–121.

Lundberg, I., Frost, J. and Petersen, O.P. (1988). Effects of an extensive program for stimulating phonological awareness in preschool children. *Reading Research Quarterly, 23,* 264–284.

Lundberg, I., Olofsson, A. and Wall, S. (1980). Reading and spelling skills in the first school years predicted from phonemic awareness skills in kindergarten. *Scandinavian Journal of Psychology, 21,* 159–173.

Marsh, G., Friedman, M.P., Welch, V. and Desberg, P. (1981). A cognitive–developmental theory of reading acquisition. In T.G. Walker and G.E. Mackinnon (Eds.), *Reading Research: Advances in Theory and Practice,* Vol. 3. London and San Diego: Academic Press.

Nicolson, R.I. and Fawcett, A.J. (1990). Automaticity: A new framework for dyslexia research? *Cognition, 35,* 159–182.

Olson, R.K., Wise, B., Conners, F., Rack, J. and Fulker, D. (1989). Specific deficits in component reading and language skills: Genetic and environmental influences. *Journal of Learning Disabilities, 22,* 339–348.

Olson, R.K., Wise, B., Conners, F. and Rack, J. (1990). Organization, hereditability, and remediation of component word recognition and language skills in disabled readers. In T.H. Carr and B.A. Levy (Eds.), *Reading and its Development: Component skills approaches*. New York: Academic Press.

Patterson, K.E. and Coltheart, V. (1987). Phonological processes in reading: A tutorial review. In M. Coltheart (Ed.), *Attention and Performance XII*. London: Erlbaum.

Patterson, K.E. and Morton, J. (1985). From orthography to phonology: an attempt at an old interpretation. In K.E. Patterson, J.C. Marshall and M. Coltheart (Eds.), *Surface Dyslexia: Neurological and cognitive studies of phonological reading*. London: Erlbaum.

Patterson, K.E., Seidenberg, M.S. and McClelland, J.L. (1989). Connections and disconnections: Acquired dyslexia in a computational model of reading processes. In R.G.M. Morris (Ed.), *Parallel Distributed Processing: Implications for psychology and neurobiology*. Oxford: Clarendon Press.

Perfetti, C.A., Beck, I., Bell, L.C. and Hughes, C. (1987). Phonemic knowledge and learning to read are reciprocal: A longitudinal study of first grade children. *Merrill–Palmer Quarterly, 33*, 283–319.

Quinlan, P. (1991). *Connectionism and Psychology*. London: Harvester Wheatsheaf.

Rayner, K., Murphy, L., Henderson, J.M. and Pollatsek, A. (1989). Selective attentional dyslexia. *Cognitive Neuropsychology, 6*, 357–378.

Rayner, K. and Pollatsek, A. (1989). *The Psychology of Reading*. London: Prentice-Hall.

Reitsma, P. (1988). Reading practice for beginners: Effects of guided reading, reading–while–listening, and independent reading with computer-based speech feedback. *Reading Research Quarterly, 23,* 219–235.

Schwartz, M.F., Saffran, E.M. and Marin, O.S.M. (1980). Fractionating the reading process in dementia. Evidence for word-specific print–to–sound association. In M. Coltheart, K. Patterson, and J. C. Marshall (Eds.), *Deep Dyslexia*. London: Routledge and Kegan Paul.

Schwartz, S. (1984). *Measuring Reading Competence: A theoretical prescriptive approach*. London: Plenum.

Seidenberg, M.S. (1985). Constraining models of word recognition. *Cognition, 20*, 169–190.

Seidenberg, M.S. and McClelland, J.L. (1989). A distributed, developmental model of word recognition and naming. *Psychological Review, 96*, 523–568.

Seymour, P.H.K. and Elder L. (1986). Beginning reading without phonology. *Cognitive Neuropsychology, 3*, 1–36.

Snowling, M.J. (1980). The development of grapheme–phoneme correspondences in normal and dyslexic readers. *Journal of Experimental Child Psychology, 29*, 294–305.

Snowling, M.J. (1981). Phonemic deficits in developmental dyslexia. *Psychological Research, 43*, 219–234.

Snowling, M.J. and Hulme, C. (1989). A longitudinal case study of developmental phonological dyslexia. *Cognitive Neuropsychology, 6*, 379–401.

Stanovich, K.E. (1986). Matthew effects in reading: Some consequences of individual differences in the acquisition of literacy. *Reading Research Quarterly, 21*, 360–406.

Stanovich, K.E. and Cunningham, A.E. (1992). Studying the consequences of literacy within a literate society: The cognitive correlates of print exposure. *Memory and Cognition, 20*, 51–68.

Stanovich, K.E. and West, R.F. (1989). Exposure to print and orthographic processing. *Reading Research Quarterly, 24*, 402–433.

Stuart, M. and Coltheart, M. (1988). Does reading develop in a sequence of stages? *Cognition, 30*, 139–181.

Taraban, R. and McClelland, J.L. (1987). Conspiracy effects in word pronunciation. *Journal of Memory and Language, 26*, 608–631.

Treiman, R., Goswami, U. and Bruck, M. (1990). Not all nonwords are alike: Implications for reading development and theory. *Memory and Cognition, 18*, 559–567.

Treiman, R. and Hirsh–Pasek, K. (1985). Are there qualitative differences in reading behavior between dyslexics and normal readers? *Memory and Cognition, 13*, 357–364.

Van Daal, V.H.P. and van der Leij, A. (1992). Computer–based reading and spelling practice for children with learning disabilities. *Journal of Learning Disabilities, 25*, 186–195.

Van Orden, G.C., Pennington, B.F. and Stone, G.O. (1990). Word identification in reading and the promise of subsymbolic psycholinguistics. (1990). *Psychological Review, 97*, 488–522.

Wagner, R.K. (1988). Causal relations between the development of phonological processing abilities and the acquisition of reading skills: A meta–analysis. *Merrill–Palmer Quarterly, 34*, 261–279.

Wagner, R.K. and Torgesen, J.K. (1987). The nature of phonological processing and its causal role in the acquisition of reading skills. *Psychological Bulletin, 101*, 192–212.

West, F.F., Madison, J. and Stanovich, K.E. (1991). The incidental acquisition of information from reading. *Psychological Science, 2*, 325–330.

Wilding, J. (1989). Developmental dyslexics do not fit in boxes: Evidence from the case studies. *European Journal of Cognitive Psychology, 1*, 105–127.

CHAPTER 3

Automaticity deficits in word reading

Regina Yap and Aryan van der Leij

INTRODUCTION

Learning to read can be described as the strengthening of connections between relevant aspects of words. These aspects involve information about orthography, phonology, meaning, syntax, articulation and grapho-motor production of words. Before children start to learn to read they already possess knowledge about meaning and articulation of words that are used frequently in everyday live. They also have some implicit knowledge about the syntactical aspects of language. Although they cannot explicitly label words as nouns or adjectives, they are capable of using the words properly within sentences.

However, it is not until reading instruction begins at school that children start to develop advanced orthographic, phonological and grapho-motor knowledge. During the course of learning to read and write the awareness of links between orthographic and phonological units are stimulated. As a result of practice, the child is able to exploit an increasing span of visual analysis. Starting from the mapping of single graphemes to single phonemes, the child is soon able to process clusters of letters and eventually whole words. Words that have been read repeatedly will be processed accurately and with increasing speed. New or unknown words will be processed at a lower level of visual analysis, which is indicated by a slower speed of word recognition and possibly, a lower degree of accuracy. When the orthographic and the phonological aspects of words are 'well-connected' word reading may be called automatic.

Automatic processing is the final stage in isolated word reading. However, it is not the final stage in the overall reading process. When words are processed automatically a solid basis is provided for reading comprehension, the ultimate goal of reading. The line of reasoning is that automatic processing requires minimal demand on the capacity of the system, hence leaving more capacity for higher-order comprehension processes. Although the measurement of the extent to which a skill is automatised is a delicate undertaking, the theoretical importance of automatism is generally acknowledged (Shiffrin, Dumais and Schneider, 1984). Automaticity is normally defined as a mode of processing that is executed rapidly, is free from demands on processing capacity, is not subject to voluntary control and is not susceptible to interruption by competing activity that interferes in the same domain (Jonides, Naveh-Benjamin and Palmer, 1985; Schneider, 1985; Shiffrin, Dumais and Schneider, 1984. See also the chapter by Fawcett and Nicolson, this volume.) Applied to the lexical domain, the automatic stage is characterised by accurate and fast reading of words, in which speed of processing reaches an asymptotic level (Laberge and Samuels, 1974; Samuels, 1985). Perfetti (1992) adds to this the notion of 'cognitive impenetrability', referring to the insensitivity of the so-called 'autonomous lexicon' to interfering stimuli or change in task demands. A word is processed autonomously when its processing is accurate and fast, time and again, irrespective of stimulus and response conditions.

Children with severe reading disabilities, the so-called dyslexics, have to put much effort in the process of word recognition and their reading development is very slow. The aim of this chapter is to investigate the issue of whether dyslexics are eventually capable of automatic word processing. To examine automatic processing, we disturbed the reading process by putting a time constraint on input processing by means of a flashed format presentation of single words under short exposure durations. If word processing is automatised, performance in the constrained condition (speeded reading task) should be accurate and should not differ very much from the unconstrained condition (unspeeded reading task). The idea is that when word processing is not susceptible to such an external manipulation in exposure duration, the lexicon operates 'autonomously' under fast execution time. In short, the lexicon operates in the automatic mode. Note that we consider that the lexicon includes not only words but also parts of words. Theoretically, such a notion keeps the possibility that pseudowords too can be processed automatically. The proposed way of measuring automaticity in reading has the advantage that the output being measured is the reading act itself. This is in contrast to other automaticity measures like performances on picture-word interference tasks, in which the act of picture naming is taken as an indirect measure of reading or decoding automaticity.

In three studies, we investigated how accurately dyslexics can read words aloud on unspeeded and speeded reading tasks. In each study the dyslexics were about 10 years old and had a reading lag of at least two years. We looked at their current performance level (study 1), their rate of progress (study 2), and their sensitivity to intervention (study 3). In the first two studies the performance of dyslexics was compared with that of reading-age controls. In the third study, the effect of two computer-assisted training programs on the reading ability of dyslexics was investigated. The combination of results of the cross-sectional, longitudinal and instructional studies allows us to investigate the question whether the reading problem of dyslexics is subject to a persistent, hard to overcome deficit or a developmental lag.

STUDY 1: AUTOMATICITY OF WORD AND PSEUDOWORD READING

In this study, we examined the automaticity of word and pseudoword reading in dyslexics at the most simple level of word structure, that is the level of CVC words and CVC pseudowords. Two different naming tasks were used: an unspeeded and a speeded version. In the unspeeded version, words remained on a screen until the subject responded. In the speeded version, words remained on the screen for only 200 ms, terminated by a mask. It is assumed that impaired performance in the speeded naming task is the consequence of vulnerability of the lexicon to external manipulation, which results in insufficient time to process the word before the arrival of the mask. Hence, performance in the speeded naming task reflects the state of automaticity. A reading level-match design was used to decide whether problems found in dyslexics were subject to a specific deficit or a developmental lag. Since this design is a central point in this and the next study, the rationale for including the various control groups will be described briefly. For a detailed description of this study see Yap and van der Leij (1993).

In the current design, dyslexics were matched with three groups: (1) normal readers of the same age, (2) normal readers of the same reading level, and (3) poor readers of the same reading level. The poor readers lagged only a half year up to one year behind in reading, in contrast to the reading lag of dyslexics which was at least two years behind expectation. Because of the aberrant reading profile of dyslexics, it is important to decide on which aspect of reading dyslexics are matched with reading-age controls (for a recent review on this subject see Rack, Snowling and Olson, 1992). In this study, subjects were matched on speeded reading of words in a continuous-trial word task, a task in which words were presented in a list. In the experimental tasks, by contrast, discrete-trial reading tasks were used to test single word processing. Several authors (e.g., Bowers and Swanson, 1991; Spring and Davis, 1988; Stanovich, 1981; Wolf, 1986) suggest that discrete-trial reading tasks tap the lower, automatic reading processes better than the continuous-trial reading tasks. In the latter, more strategic processing is allowed in the form of compensating low accuracy with high speed and vice versa, or partially processing the next word while the current word is still being processed. By matching dyslexics with reading-age controls on a continuous-trial reading task and comparing them experimentally on isolated word processing, we can investigate whether dyslexics have a deficit in the lower, automatic processes of reading in particular. The argument in favour of a deficit will be strongest if dyslexics have a pattern of performance that is below reading-age level as well as below age level. Furthermore, if dyslexics differ in this way from poor readers, support is provided for the viewpoint that dyslexia is a unique disorder that differs from other types of less skilled reading.

Method

Subjects

All groups were tested in May/June, at the end of the school year. See Table 3.1 for subject characteristics. Twenty-one dyslexics in the age range of 9 to 11 years were selected from a special school for primary learning disabled children. These children had severe reading and spelling problems which could not be accounted for by factors such as intelligence; home or school background; neurological, sensory or emotional disturbance. (For a further description of the Dutch system of Special Education, see van der Leij, 1987.) The reading-age controls (RA), poor readers (Poor), and chronological-age controls (CA) were recruited from two regular schools.

To match the dyslexic group with the two reading-age groups, a Dutch reading task, called the EMT, was used (Brus and Voeten, 1973). The EMT is a standardised measure of speeded word reading and has a high reliability ($R = 0.89$). The test requires the child to read within 1 minute a list of unrelated words; the reading rate is the number of words correctly read aloud within the minute. In Table 3.1, the EMT scores are presented in words per minute (wpm), with the reading-grade equivalents shown in the next column. The Peabody Picture Vocabulary Test (PPVT) was used to test receptive vocabulary (shown in Table 3.1 as PPVT IQ scores). There were no significant differences between groups on this IQ measure.

Tasks

1. Unspeeded naming task: subjects read aloud words and pseudowords which remained on the screen until the subject responded.
2. Speeded naming task: subjects read aloud words and pseudowords which were exposed for only 200 ms.

Table 3.1 Subject characteristics in study 1

Groups	N	Age (in months)	EMT (in wpm*)	Reading grade equivalent	PPVT IQ
RA	16	85(3.96)	24.4 (7.89)	2.1	96.4 (14.4)
Poor	15	98(3.48)	29.6 (7.73)	2.4	99.6 (18.9)
Dyslexic	21	122(8.04)	27.7 (6.81)	2.3	109.0 (14.1)
CA	15	121(8.64)	64.2 (12.1)	4.6	109.0 (12.5)

Notes
*wpm = words per minute.
  The numbers within brackets are standard deviations.

Procedure

Subjects were instructed to read aloud the words as quickly and accurately as possible. Error rates were scored by hand. The stimuli were presented in discrete-trial format on an Apple Macintosh micro computer. The words were presented in lower-case characters, with point size 48, and a proportional font comparable to the font used in Dutch reading books at school.

The onset of a trial was preceded by a frame which was as large as the length and width of the word that was about to appear in it. After the word was displayed within its frame, removal of the word depended on the condition in which the word was presented. In the unspeeded condition, frame plus word were removed from the monitor by the onset of a response. In the speeded condition, the word disappeared after 200 ms and was replaced by a backward-masking stimulus, a nonsense pattern that consisted of partial features of letters (i.e. circles and lines). The mask was displayed within the same frame as the word for a period of 200 ms Afterwards, the masking stimulus disappeared and an empty frame was left which was removed at the onset of the subject's response. The subjects were instructed that the onset of their own responses terminated the frame display. After a response was made, a 3-second delay followed until the warning tone announcing the next stimulus appeared. The unspeeded condition always preceded the speeded condition.

Eighty words were presented, 40 high-frequency CVC words and 40 CVC pseudowords, equally divided across unspeeded and speeded conditions, and presented in 4 blocks of 20 trials. After a block of 20 trials, a 10-second rest was taken. Each block contained a mixed list of half high-frequency words and half pseudowords, presented in random order.

Results

The results for percentage correct are shown in Figure 3.1. It is apparent that the dyslexic group are specifically impaired in the speeded pseudoword condition.

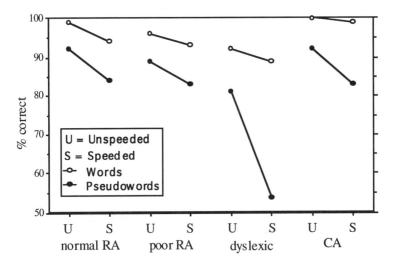

Figure 3.1 Word and pseudoword reading as a function of time constraint in the four groups

The data were subjected to a three-factor analysis of variance. Group (4 levels) was the between-subjects factor. The within-subjects variables were exposure-duration (unspeeded vs. speeded) and lexicality (words vs. pseudowords). All main effects and all possible combinations of effects were significant. There was a significant three-way interaction between group, exposure duration and lexicality [$F(3,63) = 7.17$, $p \leq .001$]. The interaction can best be interpreted as evidence that dyslexics were relatively more impaired in pseudoword reading in the speeded condition. Analyses of the interaction, taking separate Newman-Keuls *post-hoc* analyses for each combination of exposure duration and lexicality, showed that the dyslexic group made significantly more errors than the three control groups, whereas the control groups did not differ significantly from each other. In other words, the dyslexic group made significantly more errors than the control groups in reading words and pseudowords in both the unspeeded and the speeded condition.

There was also a significant interaction between group and exposure duration in the reading of pseudowords [$F(3,63) = 7.84$, $p \leq .001$], but not in the reading of the high-frequency words. There was also a significant interaction between group and lexicality in the speeded condition [$F(3,63) = 7.84$, $p \leq .001$], but not in the unspeeded condition. The interactions show that pseudoword reading of dyslexics was very much more impaired than that of the remaining groups in the speeded condition though not in the unspeeded condition.

Regression analyses

Stepwise regression analyses were run to investigate to what extent, in each group, continuous reading (EMT) was predicted by performances on each of the discrete-trial reading tasks. Vocabulary scores (PPVT) were entered as a control variable at the first step and each of the discrete reading measures at a second step. Four predictors were used in separate analyses: (1) unspeeded reading of words, (2) unspeeded reading of pseudowords, (3) speeded reading of words, and (4) speeded reading of pseudowords. The results are presented in Table 3.2 (adjusted R^2 values are reported). The motivation for doing the analyses was the above-mentioned finding that dyslexics differed from reading-age controls on discrete-trial reading tasks, whereas they performed equally on the continuous reading task (EMT) on which they were matched.

Table 3.2 shows different results for different groups. In the dyslexic group, none of the discrete reading measures contributed significantly to continuous reading. In the other groups, on the contrary, continuous reading was explained by discrete reading, but the type of discrete reading performance that contributed significantly to continuous reading was different for each group. After controlling for variance contributed by vocabulary scores, significant amounts of variance in continuous reading were predicted by unspeeded pseudoword reading in the RA group (29%), speeded pseudoword reading in the poor readers (37%) and speeded word reading in the CA group (35%).

Table 3.2 Predicting continuous reading performance from discrete reading measures

Group	Variable	Continuous Reading (EMT)		
		Step	R	R^2-adj
RA	PPVT IQ	1	0.13	−0.05
	Unspeeded word	2	0.48	0.11
	Unspeeded pseudoword	2	0.62	0.29*
	Speeded word	2	0.55	0.19
	Speeded pseudoword	2	0.53	0.17
Poor	PPVT IQ	1	0.01	−0.08
	Unspeeded word	2	0.16	−0.14
	Unspeeded pseudoword	2	0.54	0.17
	Speeded word	2	0.39	0.01
	Speeded pseudoword	2	0.68	0.37*
Dyslexic	PPVT IQ	1	0.08	−0.05
	Unspeeded word	2	0.15	−0.02
	Unspeeded pseudoword	2	0.29	−0.09
	Speeded word	2	0.32	<0.01
	Speeded pseudoword	2	0.17	−0.08
CA	PPVT IQ	1	0.03	−0.08
	Unspeeded word	2	0.03	−0.17
	Unspeeded pseudoword	2	0.27	−0.08
	Speeded word	2	0.67	0.35*
	Speeded pseudoword	2	0.19	−0.12

* $p < .05$

Discussion

Although the dyslexic children had the same reading level as reading-age controls on a continuous-trial reading task, they appeared to have lower levels of isolated word and pseudoword reading, regardless of whether reading was involved in the speeded or unspeeded condition. Furthermore, dyslexics were particularly impaired in reading pseudowords in the speeded condition. This suggests that dyslexics have a deficit in automatic decoding, even at the simplest level of word structure (CVC). The deficit seems to be specific to dyslexics and does not pertain to the poor readers in the present study.

The regression analyses shed light on the aberrant reading process of dyslexics. Unlike the control groups, their skills in isolated word and pseudoword reading did not predict their continuous reading performance. As discussed earlier, reading words in a continuous list allows higher-order reading strategies, whereas reading words in discrete format forces reliance more on the lower, automatic processes of reading. The results of the regression analyses indicate that dyslexics depend on other processes than those triggered by the discrete-trial reading tasks to achieve equal levels of continuous reading performance to the reading-age controls. Probably, dyslexics make relatively more use of compensation strategies. We will return to this suggestion in the general discussion.

STUDY 2: DEVELOPMENT OF WORD READING AUTOMATICITY

Study 1 demonstrated that dyslexics have a deficit in single word processing and that they rely on atypical processes for continuous reading. Study 2 was designed to detect how these cross-sectional differences change over the course of time. The reading development of dyslexics is slow and this may be due to an atypical rate of acquisition of specific cognitive processes.

The aim of this study was to find out how dyslexics develop in accuracy and rate of word processing at increasing levels of phonological and orthographic complexity. (See p. 88 for distinguishing phonological from orthographic complexity in the Dutch language.) Again, dyslexics were matched with reading-age controls on the same continuous reading task as described in study 1. Also, the same kind of tasks (unspeeded and speeded reading tasks) were used to tap automaticity of processing. The children were tested twice. In order to equate reading levels across groups at both the initial and final tests, the period between assessments had to be longer for the dyslexics than for the reading-age controls: the interval between the two testing periods was 18.8 months for the dyslexic group and 9.2 months for the reading-age control group. This clearly demonstrates that, in a quantitative sense, the overall reading development of dyslexics is about twice as slow as that of younger, normal readers. By investigating characteristics of single word reading over the course of time, we also tried to find out whether dyslexics differ in the way they reach a particular reading level.

Method

Subjects

See Table 3.3 for subject characteristics. See study 1 for the procedure for selecting dyslexics and for matching the dyslexic group with the reading-age group. The reading-age controls (RA) were average readers who came from regular schools. The Peabody Picture Vocabulary Test (PPVT) was administered at the second testing period. The RA group had significant higher PPVT IQ scores than the dyslexic group ($p < .01$).

Table 3.3 Subject characteristics in study 2

Groups	N	Age (in months)	EMT (in wpm*)	Reading grade equivalent	PPVT IQ
First Testing					
RA	20	88 (3.10)	22.9 (8.88)	2.1	
Dyslexic	20	122 (12.0)	22.5 (8.55)	2.1	
Second Testing					
RA	20	97 (8.04)	39.9 (13.2)	2.9	115.6 (16.0)**
Dyslexic	20	140 (12.0)	36.6 (11.0)	2.8	100.7 (16.6)

Note. The numbers within brackets are standard deviations.
*wpm = words per minute
** $p < .01$

Procedure

The reading-age group was tested in June (the end of grade 1) and, after 9 months, in April (in grade 2). The dyslexic group was tested in November/December and, after 18 months, in May/June. The first testing time is referred to as t1, the second as t2.

A speeded and an unspeeded naming task were used. See study 1 for a description of the tasks. In contrast to study 1, exposure durations in the speeded condition decreased from 200 to 160 to 100 ms to increase pressure on fast word processing. Also, different word categories were used. These categories reflect different mastery levels (see following section).

The tasks were administered in separate sessions of 10 minutes. First, the unspeeded naming task was administered in blockwise order from easy to difficult word categories. Then the speeded naming task followed, in blockwise order from easy to difficult word categories and from long to short exposure durations.

In each block, 10 items were presented from one word category in one of the four formats of exposure duration (unlimited, 200 ms, 160 ms and 100 ms). The criterion for mastery was set at 90% correct answers per block. When a child failed to pass this criterion, items from next mastery levels (word categories) were not presented.

The scores on each task were presented in amounts of mastery, ranging from 0 to 100%. A 100% mastery level indicated that the child has passed all six word categories at criterion level. A 0% level indicated that the child did not master the most simple level of word category (CVC words). In the speeded reading task, mastery levels also upgraded along the exposure duration dimension. Thus, a 100% mastery level in the speeded naming task indicated complete mastery of all word categories in the most difficult condition of exposure duration (100 ms).

Materials

Six word categories of increasing phonological and orthographic complexity were used: (1) CVC words ('jas' = coat), (2) CVCC words ('kalf' = calf), (3) CCVC words ('vloer' = floor), (4) 'simple' two-syllable words ('poeder' = powder), (5) 'closed' two-syllable words ('bommen' = bombs), and (6) 'open' two-syllable words (bomen = trees). All were high-frequency words.

Since the correspondence between orthography and phonology is quite regular in the Dutch language, most of the one-syllable words do not present particular orthographic difficulties. However, double (or even triple) consonants at the beginning or end of the word contribute to phonological complexity. Therefore, the word categories 1–3 can be seen as increasing in phonological difficulty. In contrast, the two-syllable words, categories 4–6 represent different levels of orthographic complexity. Category 4 ('poeder') is the simplest level of orthographic processing because it does not contain any orthographic ambiguity other than the pronunciation of the accentless 'e' at the end. Categories 5 and 6 ('bommen', 'bomen') have a more difficult orthographic structure because the pronunciation of the first vowel has to be determined from the number of written consonants that follow. For example, in 'bommen' ('bombs'), which is a word from category 5, the vowel is short (as in the English word 'rotten') because of the double 'm'; in 'bomen' ('trees'), which is a word from category 6, the pronunciation of the 'o' is long (as in the English word 'open'), because of the single 'm'. So the orthographic complexity is greater in categories 5 and 6 than in 4.

Results

Unspeeded reading task

A 2 (group) x 2 (time of testing) ANOVA was run on mastery scores. There was a significant main effect of group [$F(1,38) = 11.2$, $p \leq .01$] and a significant main effect of time [$F(1,38) = 39.5$, $p \leq .001$]. There was no significant group x time interaction. As is illustrated in Figure 3.2, the dyslexic group performed significantly lower than the RA group at both testing times. Both groups showed a significant progression from t1 to t2. The rate of progression was equal for both groups.

Speeded reading task

A 2 (group) x 2 (time of testing) ANOVA was run on mastery scores. There was a significant group x time interaction [$F(1,38) = 8.35$, $p \leq .01$]. Analyses of the interaction showed that the dyslexic group did not differ significantly from the RA group at t1, but at t2 the RA group outperformed the dyslexic group. The progression in both groups was significant but was smaller for the dyslexic group. (See Figure 3.2.)

Effects of phonological and orthographic complexity

To give an indication of mastery differentiated along word category levels, we counted the number of subjects who passed mastery criteria along these levels. In Table 3.4, the percentages of competent readers on the unspeeded reading task are presented. The unspeeded reading task was chosen for further investigation in order to separate phonological and orthographic processing from automatic processing. As discussed above, categories 1–3 reflect increasing phonological complexity, whereas categories 4–6 indicate increasing orthographic complexity.

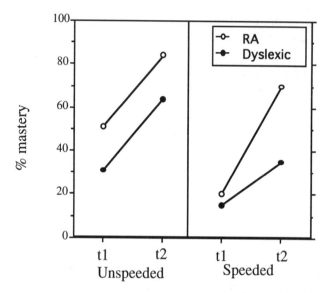

Figure 3.2 Rate of progression through the unspeeded and speeded reading tasks

Table 3.4 shows that the effect of increasing phonological complexity of one-syllable words was more dramatic in the dyslexic group than in the RA group at both testing periods (word categories 1–3). At the first assessment, both groups mastered the words with the least phonological complexity (CVC). However, only 50% of the dyslexic subjects were competent in the accurate processing of double consonants at the end of the word (CVCC), and a mere 25% could handle CCVC words. In contrast, 75% of the RA group mastered CVCC words and 65% mastered CCVC words. At the second assessment, all children from the RA group mastered the one-syllable words, independent of phonological complexity, whereas 30% of the dyslexic group were still not able to cope with CCVC words.

Table 3.4 Percentages of competent readers per word category

	Word categories					
	Increasing phonological complexity (one-syllable words)			Increasing orthographic complexity (two-syllable words)		
Group	1. CVC	2. CVCC	3. CCVC	4. simple	5. closed	6. open
First testing						
RA	100	75	65	35	35	5
Dyslexic	100	50	25	15	10	0
Second testing						
RA	100	100	100	90	85	40
Dyslexic	100	95	70	65	50	30

The effect of increasing orthographic complexity was about the same in both groups. It is important to note that, because of the word length effect, two-syllable words are more difficult to read than one-syllable words. Since the dyslexic children were less competent than the RA controls at the one-syllable level, they were also less able to read the two-syllable words. To detect an extra effect of orthographic complexity, the difference between levels of two-syllable words was investigated. The first time, most of the children in both groups did not master the two-syllable words at even the most simple level (category 4). The second time, it was clear that the category of 'open' syllables (category 6) caused both groups trouble. When categories 4 and 6 were compared, only 40% of the 90% children from the RA group who mastered category 4 could cope with the open-syllable words from category 6. In the dyslexic group, the proportion was 30% out of 65%. Thus, the drop in competence, indicated by comparison of category 4 and 6 was about the same proportionally in both groups. This result indicates that the effect of orthographic complexity was comparable in the two groups.

Effects of exposure duration
To study the effect of exposure duration, the number of subjects were counted who passed mastery criteria along the different levels of exposure duration. In Table 3.5 the results are shown, averaged over word categories.

Dyslexia in Children

Table 3.5 Percentages of competent readers per exposure duration

		exposure duration	
Group	unlimited	200 ms	100 ms
First testing			
RA	53	25	14.2
Dyslexic	33.3	28.2	4.2
Second testing			
RA	85.5	80	60
Dyslexic	68.3	55	25

The scores in the unlimited condition represent the performance in the unspeeded reading task. The unspeeded reading performance of the dyslexic group was lower than that of the RA group at both times of assessment. As we saw in the previous section, this was probably due to the effect of phonological complexity.

The scores in the 200 and 100 ms conditions represent the performance in the speeded reading task. The scores in the 160 ms condition were omitted because the scores decreased in a linear way from the 200 to the 160 and the 100 ms condition. Table 3.5 shows that at the first testing period, the dyslexic and the RA groups were comparable at the 200 ms level: most of them failed. In the 100 ms condition, the RA group performed slightly better than the dyslexic group. At the second testing period, differences between the two groups, in favour of the RA group, showed up at all levels of limited exposure duration.

To give an indication of the effects of demand on automatic processing, we looked at the difference between speeded and unspeeded reading at t2. Averaged over word categories, the proportion of competent normal readers dropped from 85.8% (unlimited condition) to 80% (200 ms) to 60% (100 ms). In the dyslexic group, the proportion decreased from 68.3% to 55% to 25%. So the difference between dyslexics and reading-age controls increased cumulatively as more demand was made on automatic processing.

Regression analyses
For each testing period, the amount of variance in continuous reading contributed by discrete reading performance was computed

by regression analyses. Again, vocabulary scores (PPVT) were entered at the first step. Since there were no PPVT IQ scores available at the first testing period, we used the IQ scores of the second assessment to enter the first step in regression at t1. At the second step, two predictors were used in separate analyses: (1) unspeeded reading across word categories, and (2) speeded reading across word categories. Table 3.6 shows the results.

The results showed that at t1, after controlling for variance contributed by vocabulary scores, significant amounts of variance in continuous reading were predicted by speeded reading at the single word level, both in the RA group (69%) and in the dyslexic group (51%). In the dyslexic group, unspeeded reading at the single word level also contributed to continuous reading (38%). A striking finding is the high correlation found in the dyslexic group between PPVT IQ and the continuous reading measure (EMT). Notice, however, that the correlation between vocabulary and continuous reading is negatively loaded. Entered at the first step, PPVT IQ predicted a significant 28% of the total amount of variance in dyslexics' continuous reading. In contrast, PPVT IQ of the RA group did not predict reading on the EMT.

Table 3.6 Predicting continuous reading performance (EMT) from unspeeded and speeded reading measures

Group	Variable	Step	Continuous Reading t1		Continuous Reading t2	
			R	R^2-adj	R	R^2-adj
RA	PPVT IQ	1	0.14	−0.04	0.14	−0.04
	Unspeeded	2	0.50	0.16	0.64	0.35**
	Speeded	2	0.85	0.69**	0.77	0.54**
Dyslexic	PPVT IQ	1	−0.56	0.28**	−0.48	0.19*
	Unspeeded	2	0.67	0.38**	0.49	0.15
	Speeded	2	0.75	0.51***	0.58	0.26

$* p < .05$ $** p < .01$ $*** p < .001$

At the second assessment, discrete reading measures contribute significantly to continuous reading only in the RA group (35% by unspeeded reading and, analysed separately, 54% by speeded reading). None of the discrete reading measures added significant amounts of variance to the continuous reading performances of dyslexics, after controlling for variance contributed by vocabulary scores. In contrast, a significant amount of variance was explained by vocabulary IQ scores (19%).

Discussion

In study 2, a developmental perspective was taken to investigate whether dyslexics differed from reading-age controls in the way they reach the same global level of reading performance. Indeed, dyslexics were slower in reading development because they took twice as long as reading-age controls to reach equivalent scores in reading continuous words. This study provides evidence that atypical processing underlies the slow reading development of dyslexics for three reasons.

In the first place, dyslexics progressed significantly slower than reading-age controls in speeded reading despite a similar progression profile in unspeeded reading (Figure 3.2). Only 25% of the dyslexic children could, at the age of 12, process the words fast enough in the 100 ms condition, against 60% of the normal readers at the age of 8 (Table 3.5). Furthermore, dyslexics were progressively more affected by shortening the exposure durations compared to reading-age controls. These results suggest that dyslexics have an atypical rate of acquisition of the automatic skills needed for reading in constrained conditions.

Second, despite similar progression profiles in unspeeded reading, dyslexics performed below reading-age level at both times of assessment. Probably, this is due to specific problems with the processing of phonological features of words rather than orthographic ones (Table 3.4). At a time when all reading-age controls had mastered phonologically complex CCVC words with double consonants in the initial position, 30% of the dyslexics were still not able to cope with CCVC words. Apart from the observation that dyslexics performed worse than reading-age controls in all word categories, there was no evidence that they were particularly impaired in reading words with increasing orthographic complexity. In sum, the results suggest that dyslexics have a deficit in phonological processing.

A third indication of idiosyncratic processing in dyslexics was provided by the regression analyses. The results for their continuous reading suggest that as development progresses, dyslexics rely increasingly on processes other than those necessary for single word processing. The significant amount of variance explained by vocabulary IQ scores suggests that dyslexic readers rely on semantic knowledge in their word reading. However, their vocabulary was inversely related to their reading performance. This finding rather appeals to the foundation construct in the definition of dyslexia reflecting a discrepancy between aptitude and achievement (Stanovich, 1991).

In conclusion, the results of study 2 support the deficit hypothesis of dyslexia. Dyslexics seem to have an atypical rate of acquisition of two specific cognitive processes needed in single word reading. First, they were particularly slow in acquiring automatic skills and, second, they were particularly slow in acquiring knowledge of the phonological properties of words. Furthermore, regression analyses suggest that, during development, dyslexics rely increasingly on atypical processes for reading to compensate for their deficit.

STUDY 3: TRAINING IN READING AUTOMATICITY

The cross-sectional study (study 1) showed that dyslexics have particular problems with rapid processing of pseudowords. Pseudoword reading requires decoding of the word into sublexical units; the translation of orthographic units into phonological units is an important part in this process. Combined with problems in speed of processing, demonstrated in the cross-sectional and the longitudinal study (studies 1 and 2), the problem of dyslexics can be described as an impairment in making fast grapheme–phoneme correspondences at the sublexical level (see also the chapter by Beech in this volume).

Another research strategy is to use intervention techniques to investigate reading problems (Backman, Mamen, and Ferguson, 1984; Bradley and Bryant, 1985). The aim of the present study was to examine whether dyslexics can improve their word and pseudoword reading by increasing the speed of decoding at the sublexical level. The rationale of the intervention study is that if dyslexics have an intractable deficit in fast decoding, training of the defective component will not lead to substantive transfer to pseudoword reading. The training is a computer-assisted program known as the speed-decoding training. For a detailed description of this study, see Yap (1993).

Method

Design and general procedure

A pre-test–training–post-test design was used, comparing performance of dyslexic children trained on the speed decoding program with that of a matched control group of dyslexic children who also received intensive word training on the computer but were not specifically trained in fast processing of sublexical units (see Training tasks below). By comparing the experimental speed-decoding training with the control word training, the influence of extraneous factors such as individual attention, intensive instruction and group characteristics were excluded.

The children were trained three times a week for a period of 10 minutes a day. The total amount of training time was 160 minutes for both the experimental and the control group.

Subjects

See Table 3.7 for subject characteristics. The experimental and the control group consisted of dyslexics who were matched on age and reading level on the EMT (see study 1 for a description of the EMT). They were selected in the same manner as described previously in study 1.

Training tasks

1. Speed-decoding training. The instructional setting of the training is derived from the perceptual-unit training of Frederiksen, Warren and Roseberry (1985). However, in this training program, the modality of presenting the sublexical unit differed in that a spoken phoneme cluster was presented to the child through headphones and a visual word was presented on a computer screen. The child had to press a 'yes' button when the sound of the phoneme cluster was

within the word and a 'no' button when it was absent. Thus, the child had to make a correspondence between phonemic and orthographic units. By gradually shortening the exposure duration of the written word, dependent on accuracy of performance, the child was stimulated to enhance his or her speed of processing. In total, 10 different phoneme clusters were presented 8 times repeatedly, with words sampled from a database of 2021 one-to-three-syllable words.

Table 3.7 Subject characteristics in study 3

Training	N	Age (in months)	EMT (in wpm *)	Reading grade equivalent
Speed-decoding	19	124.4 (10.0)	26.8 (10.0)	2.3
Control	22	121.5 (9.5)	27.7 (7.3)	2.3

Note. Numbers within brackets are standard deviations.
* wpm = words per minute

2. Control training. The control training was an existing instructional program, called COPAL (van Daal *et al.* 1987). COPAL consists of a variety of reading and spelling tasks but is not specifically aimed at fast processing of sublexical units.

Pre- and post-tests
1. EMT: see study 1.
    2. Unspeeded reading task. See study 1 for the general procedure, but different material was used and this time response latency was also measured, by means of a voice key. Each stimulus was sampled without replacement from a set of 20 words and 20 pseudowords, and remained on the screen until the subject responded. The words had a simple two-syllable structure (category 4 in study 2) and the pseudowords had a CVCC or a CCVC structure.
    3. Speeded reading task. See study 1 for the general procedure. Each stimulus was sampled without replacement from a set of 20 words and 20 pseudowords, and was presented for a period of 200 ms. The material was different from that in the unspeeded reading task but the word structures were the same.

Results

1. Continuous reading task (EMT). A 2 (group) x 2 (time: pre-test vs. post-test) ANOVA showed a significant group x time interaction [$F(1,39) = 4.44$, $p \leq .05$]. As Figure 3.3 illustrates, both training groups did improve their continuous reading performance but the improvement was greater for the speed-decoding group.

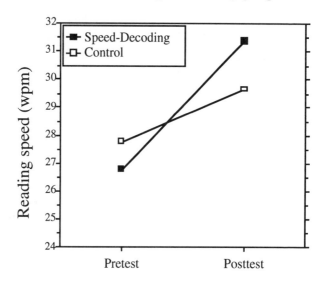

Figure 3.3 The effect of intervention on the continuous reading task (EMT)

2. Unspeeded reading task. A 2 (group) x 2 (time) x 2 (lexicality: words vs. pseudowords) ANOVA was computed on percentage correct responses and response latencies. On the accuracy data, no effects were found other than a main effect of lexicality [$F(1,39) = 27.9$, $p \leq .001$]. Words were read more accurately than pseudowords. Across times, the average percentage correct responses was 90.1% for words (SD = 11.7) and 81.5% for pseudowords (SD = 15.4).

On the response latency data, there was a main effect of time [$F(1,39) = 4.72$, $p \leq .05$], indicating that both groups did improve their reading speed. There was also a marginally significant time x lexicality interaction [$F(1,39) = 3.35$, $p = .08$]. In the pre-test, word latency for both groups was around 2500 ms for both words and pseudowords. At the post-test, the improvement in word reading speed was greater than that in pseudoword reading speed: word latency decreased by 342 ms, against a decrease of 113 ms in pseudoword latency. This holds for both groups.

3. Speeded reading task. Percentage correct responses were subjected to a 2 (group) x 2 (time) x 2 (lexicality) ANOVA. There was a main effect of time $[F(1,39) = 33.6, p \leq .001]$, which indicated that both training groups improved their speeded word and pseudoword reading. There was also a main effect of lexicality $[F(1,39) = 61.5, p \leq .001]$. Instead of the commonly found word superiority effect, there was better performance for pseudoword reading than for word reading. It is very likely that this discrepancy was caused by the greater length of the word stimuli than the pseudowords. There was similar improvement in reading for both types of stimuli, with word reading improving from 36.1% correct responses (SD = 21.8) to 48.8% (SD = 27.4), and pseudoword reading improving from 59.8% (SD = 21.4) to 66.6% (SD = 21.8).

Discussion

Study 3 showed that dyslexics can improve their reading speed on continuous and discrete reading tasks. Accuracy of unspeeded reading performance did not improve but was already high before training started.

Only on the continuous reading task was the speed-decoding training more effective than the control training (Figure 3.3). On the discrete reading tasks, the progress was similar for both groups. This suggests that a specific characteristic of the training in fast decoding is its transfer to a better use of higher-order reading processes, used in continuous reading.

Despite longer word length, words were read more accurately and faster than pseudowords. This word superiority effect is a common phenomenon in human information processing (e.g., Broadbent, 1967). However, when words were exposed for only 200 ms, dyslexics made more errors in reading the two-syllable words than the one-syllable pseudowords. In such a constrained condition, word length apparently overrules lexical facilitation in dyslexics' reading. Nevertheless, dyslexics had more difficulty processing pseudowords than words in that their response latency for word reading was more sensitive to improvement by training than their pseudoword latency.

The relatively minor improvement in pseudoword reading suggests a deficit in decoding speed. It corresponds to the notion that a deficit is hard to remedy. However, the differential effect of intervention on lexicality was not observed in the speeded reading task, which also taps reading speed. This result may be accounted for by similarity in task conditions. In the speed-decoding training and, to some extent, in the control training as well, children were trained to read words in flashed presentation format, a format that is also used in the speeded reading task. It may be that the flashed format stimulates the children to replace their time-consuming strategy by a strategy of fast visual analysis which also transfers to pseudoword reading.

In conclusion, during a short training period, dyslexics can benefit from word practice to improve reading speed without loss of accuracy. Transfer to pseudoword reading is small compared with the transfer to word reading. Training that is specifically aimed at increasing decoding speed also transfers to the higher reading processes used in continuous reading.

GENERAL DISCUSSION

In three studies, we investigated the question whether dyslexics are able to process words in a fast, facile, effortless, automatised way. Automatic word processing forms the basis for better reading: because of its minimal demands on processing capacity, more capacity is left for higher-order reading processes used for reading comprehension. To examine whether dyslexics are capable of automatic word processing, we disturbed the reading process by putting time constraints on input processing, using a flashed format presentation of the stimuli. If word processing is automatised, performance in the constrained condition (speeded reading) will be accurate and will not differ very much from the unconstrained condition (unspeeded reading). The idea is that when word processing is not susceptible to such an external manipulation in exposure duration, the lexicon operates 'autonomously' under fast execution time, or in other words, automatically.

All three studies provide evidence that dyslexics have a deficit in automatic phonological decoding. The cross-sectional study (study

1) showed that dyslexics were more susceptible to time constraints than normal and poor reading control groups when CVC pseudowords had to be processed. The longitudinal study (study 2) replicated the findings of study 1 with regard to the processing of words across various levels of word complexity. In addition, the longitudinal study revealed that dyslexics develop more slowly than reading-age controls in the time-constrained condition, despite a similar pattern of progression in the unconstrained condition. This suggests that dyslexics have an atypical rate of acquisition of automatic skills needed for speeded reading in the constrained condition. The longitudinal study also demonstrated that, as well as their problems in the constrained condition, dyslexics have relatively more problems with words that increase in phonological complexity than words that increase in orthographic complexity. This gives further evidence that the deficit is phonological in nature, in addition to problems with automatic processing. The intervention study (study 3) provided evidence that, despite intensive training in decoding speed, dyslexics were limited in their ability to improve speed of pseudoword processing compared to word processing. This suggests that the decoding deficit is hard to remedy. By contrast, the dyslexics' word reading was sensitive to intervention and the training in rapid decoding transferred to processes used in continuous reading. Theoretically, this is an interesting finding. By improving decoding speed, it may be that less demand is made on the system capacity so that more is left for strategic processing, triggered by the continuous reading task.

The results support the phonological deficit hypothesis of dyslexia (e.g., Olson *et al.*, 1985; Rack, Snowling and Olson, 1992; Snowling, 1987; see also Rack, this volume). The reading problem of dyslexics is clearly phonological by nature, indicated by relatively weak performances in reading pseudowords (studies 1 and 3) and phonologically complex words (study 2). There is evidence that the phonological deficit is fairly independent of other deficits because it occurred in conditions where no further complicated task demands were required (study 2). However, there is also evidence that the phonological problem of dyslexics was worst in conditions where strong demand is made on automatic processing (studies 1 and 2). This suggests that dyslexics have at least one other deficit as well as the phonological one. As far as reading is concerned, the results fit the automatisation deficit hypothesis of Nicolson and

Fawcett (1990). The hypothesis claims that dyslexia is caused by an impairment in automatic processing as a general principle of skill acquisition (see also the chapter by Fawcett and Nicolson in this volume). Consequently, the hypothesis predicts that dyslexics will have problems on every domain where automatic processing is required. The studies reported here indicate that the hypothesis holds at least for the phonological domain. Another part of the automatisation deficit hypothesis is the notion of 'conscious compensation', which states that dyslexics can reach a normal level of performance simply by 'working harder'. We regard the notion of compensation as the theoretical counterpart of the deficit concept. Empirically, our results give some support to the possibility of compensatory processing. Since, in the literature, relatively little attention is paid to the compensation concept, in contrast to the deficit concept, we will discuss the possibility of compensatory processing at some length.

The studies reported here suggest that dyslexics rely on compensation processes or strategies. Our evidence is first that dyslexics, despite equal levels of *continuous* reading performance, have lower *discrete* reading performance than reading-age controls (study 1 and 2). This indicates, on the one hand, that dyslexics have a deficit in the lower order, automatic processes tapped by isolated word reading. On the other hand, it suggests that they use different ways to come to the same reading level as reading-age controls. Second, the continuous reading performance of dyslexics is not predicted by their discrete reading performance, unlike that of the normal and poor readers (study 1). Moreover, the longitudinal study (study 2) indicates that this phenomenon becomes more marked as reading development progresses. These results suggest that dyslexics, in their general reading development, rely less and less on the basic, automatic processes that are so necessary in isolated word reading. The possibility is raised that dyslexics use strategies to compensate for their decoding deficit when task demands allow for such strategies.

Different ways of compensation are suggested by our findings. At the least, it seems to be useful to distinguish between strategies used in continuous reading and strategies used in isolated word reading. Because of the different task procedures, the former gives opportunities to make use of strategies that are not possible in isolated reading, such as compensating high accuracy with low speed and vice versa, correcting reading errors, and overlapping different stages in reading by simultaneously processing words that are next in the list or in the sentence. However, in single word reading, compensation is also possible. For instance, the presence of an aberrant developmental profile on the speeded reading task and the absence of it on the unspeeded reading task (study 2) suggests that compensatory processing, used by the dyslexics on the unspeeded task, is relatively time-consuming. Thus, the absence of time pressure is important to elicit compensation strategies. Similarly, the relatively better processing of orthographic information as opposed to phonological information (study 2) may indicate that the deficit in phonological processing is compensated for by orthographic processing. Lastly, the relatively better improvement in word reading compared to pseudoword reading, as an effect of intervention (study 3), suggests that lexical facilitation is used to compensate for the decoding deficit.

Note, however, that putting different labels on different aspects of task performance does not necessarily mean that different compensation processes or different defective mechanisms are in use. For instance, compensation by lexical facilitation may simply mean compensation by orthographic processing. Because of the higher frequency of occurrence in the written language, word reading allows more opportunity for orthographic processing than does pseudoword reading.

Whatever the nature of the compensation process(es), the studies reported here imply that compensation is related to effortful, time-consuming processing. This is reflected in the slowness of the developmental course as well as in the slowness of the information processing system. Dyslexics have to put much effort into the process of learning to read. They have to see the orthographic structure of words over and over again in order to use it, in the long run, as a way of compensating for the phonological deficit. They need more time to reach a particular reading level in development and they need more processing time to read isolated words. It is important to re-emphasise here that the parallel progression line on the unspeeded reading task in Figure 3.3 (study 2) does not mean that dyslexics progress at a similar rate to reading-age controls. The interval time between assessments was still twice as long for the dyslexic group as for the reading-age group, indicating that dyslexics develop at least twice as slowly as normal readers.

Theoretically, the opposite of compensatory characteristics reflects the nature of the defective mechanism(s). Thus, the inability to process effortlessly and fast seems to characterise the deficit in dyslexic readers. Another way of denoting to this problem is to speak in terms of an inability to process automatically. We regard both the possibilities of an automatisation deficit and of strategic compensation as important perspectives for further research.

Lastly, we would like to make some suggestions for the field of assessment and remedial practice. The assessment of children with severe reading disability should include discrete reading tasks in addition to continuous reading tasks. Isolated word reading taps the lower-order reading processes better than continuous reading and, hence, touches directly the core of the problem. Next, a reading profile is desirable to uncover particular patterns of strengths and weaknesses exhibited by dyslexic readers. Particularly, discrepancies between word vs. pseudoword processing on the one hand, and speeded vs. unspeeded reading on the other, seem to make sense for better diagnosis.

The theoretical distinction between defective mechanisms and compensatory processing leaves remedial practice free to tackle each of these two aspects separately. Focusing on the relatively weak skills suggests the use of training programmes that enhance the speed of decoding. Study 3 gave some indications that such a training can improve reading speed. An approach aimed at improvement of the relatively strong skills teaches children to use compensation strategies. For example, verbal practice with words before confronting the children with the orthographic structure seems to elicit lexical facilitation and repeated unspeeded word reading (van der Leij and van Daal, 1989a and b). Naturally, a good remedial program should focus on both the weak and the strong skills.

REFERENCES

Backman, J.E., Mamen, M. and Ferguson, H.B. (1984). Reading level design: Conceptual and methodological issues in reading research. *Psychological Bulletin*, 96, 560–568.

Bowers, P.G. and Swanson, L.B. (1991). Naming speed deficits in reading disability: Multiple measures of single processes. *Journal of Experimental Child Psychology, 51,* 195–219.

Bradley, L. and Bryant, P.E. (1985). *Rhyme and Reason in Reading and Spelling.* Ann Arbor: University of Michigan Press.

Broadbent, D.E. (1967). Word-frequency effect and response bias. *Psychological Review, 74,* 1–15.

Brus, B.T. and Voeten, M.J.M. (1973). *Een–minuuttest, vorm A en B.* Nijmegen: Berkhout.

Frederiksen, J.R., Warren, B.M. and Roseberry, A.S. (1985). A componential approach to training reading skills: Part 1. Perceptual units training. *Cognition and Instruction, 2,* 91–130.

Jonides, J., Naveh–Benjamin, M. and Palmer, J. (1985). Assessing automaticity. *Acta Psychologica, 60,* 157–171.

LaBerge, D. and Samuels, S.J. (1974). Toward a theory of automatic information processing in reading. *Cognitive Psychology, 6,* 293–323.

Manis, F.R. (1985). Acquisition of word identification skills in normal and disabled readers. *Journal of Educational Psychology, 77,* 78–90.

Nicolson, R.I. and Fawcett, A.J. (1990). Automaticity: A new framework for dyslexia research? *Cognition, 35,* 159–182.

Olson, R., Kliegl, R., Davidson, B. and Foltz, G. (1985). Individual and developmental differences in reading disability. In T. Waller (Ed.), *Reading Research: Advances in theory and practice, 4* (pp. 1–64). London: Academic Press.

Perfetti, C.A. (1992). The representation problem in reading acquisition. In P.B. Gough, L. Ehri and R. Treiman (Eds.), *Reading Acquisition.* Hillsdale, NJ: Lawrence Erlbaum.

Perfetti, C.A., Finger, E. and Hogaboam, T. (1978). Sources of vocalization latency differences between skilled and less skilled young readers. *Journal of Educational Psychology, 67,* 461–469.

Rack, J.P., Snowling, M.J. and Olson, R.K. (1992). The nonword reading deficit in developmental dyslexia: A review. *Reading Research Quarterly, 27,* 28–53.

Samuels, J. (1985). Automaticity and repeated reading. In P.T.J. Osborn, R. Wilson, and R.C. Anderson (Eds.), *Reading Education: Foundations for a literate America.* Lexington: Lexington Books.

Schneider, W. (1985). Toward a model of attention and the development of automatic processing. In M.I. Posner and O.S. Marin (Eds.), *Attention and Performance XI* (pp. 475–492). Hillsdale, NJ: Lawrence Erlbaum.

Shiffrin, R.M., Dumais, S.T. and Schneider, W. (1984). Characteristics of automatism. In J. Long and A. Baddeley (Eds.), *Attention and Performance IX.* (pp. 223–238). Hillsdale, NJ: Lawrence Erlbaum.

Snowling, M. (1987). *Dyslexia: A cognitive developmental perspective.* Oxford: Basil Blackwell.

Spring, C. and Davis, J.M. (1988). Relations of digit naming speed with three components of reading. *Applied Psycholinguistics*, *9*, 315–334.

Stanovich, K.E. (1981). Relationships between word decoding speed, general name retrieval ability, and reading progress in first-grade children. *Journal of Educational Psychology*, *73*, 809–815.

Stanovich. K.E. (1991). Discrepancy definitions of reading disability: Has intelligence led us astray? *Reading Research Quarterly*, *26* , 7–29.

Van Daal, V.H.P., van der Leij, A., Bakker, N.C.M. and Reitsma, P. (1987). Een computergestuurd orthodidactisch programma voor aanvankelijk lezen: COPAL. *Pedagogische Studiën*, *64*, pp. 364–376. (A computer–assisted program for initial reading).

Van der Leij, A. (1987). Netherlands: Special Education in the. In C.R Reynolds and L. Mann (Eds.), *Encyclopedia of Special Education* (pp. 1094–1095). New York: John Wiley and Sons.

Van der Leij, A. and Daal, V.v. (1989a). Attacking dyslexia: The effect of preceding and simultaneous verbal practice. In J.J. Dumont, and H. Nakken (Eds.), *Learning Disabilities. Vol. 2: Cognitive, social and remedial aspects*. Lisse: Swets and Zeitlinger.

Van der Leij, A. and Daal, V.v. (1989b). Repeated reading and severe reading disability. In H. Mandl, E. de Corte, N. Bennett, and H.P. Friedrich (Eds.), *Learning and Instruction (European research in an international context. Analysis of complex skills and complex knowledge domains 2.2)* (pp. 235–252). Oxford: Pergamon Press.

Wolf, M. (1986). Rapid alternative naming in the developmental dyslexias. *Brain and Language*, *27*, 360–379.

Yap, R.L. (1993). *Automatic Word Processing Deficits in Dyslexia: Qualitative differences and specific remediation*. Unpublished doctoral dissertation: Vrije Universiteit, Amsterdam.

Yap, R.L. and van der Leij, A. (1993). Word processing in dyslexics: An automatic decoding deficit? *Reading and Writing: An Interdisciplinary Journal*, *5*, 261–279.

PART 2

Visual skill, motor skill and speed of processing

The pioneers of dyslexia research, such as James Hinshelwood and Samuel Orton, believed that visual problems underlay the reading problems suffered by dyslexic children. Despite occasional demonstrations of visual anomalies, subsequent research failed to substantiate these views, leading to a general belief that 'extensive evaluation suggests that visual deficits are unlikely to be the cause of most cases of dyslexia' (Just and Carpenter, 1987, *The Psychology of Reading and Language Comprehension*, Newton, MS: Allyn and Bacon, p. 385). However, recent direct investigations of visual skill in Britain, Australia and the United States have led to striking findings of subtle visual deficits related to rapid processing of visual information, and to findings of decreased binocular stability.

The chapters in Part 2 provide overviews of the research in both these areas, with Bill Lovegrove reviewing the research on the deficits in transient visual processing (much of it undertaken in his laboratory in Wollongong, Australia), and John Stein presenting evidence from his group in Oxford on instability of binocular control in dyslexic children, again interpreting the results in terms of problems in the transient visual system. The authors suggest that the deficits in visual skill may be part of a more general impairment in temporal aspects of sensory and motor performance.

In Chapter 4, Lovegrove presents an accessible overview of a series of experiments into vision and dyslexia, arguing for a particular deficit in the transient system in dyslexics which cannot be attributed to their failure to learn to read. He first describes the two systems: the *transient system* mediates the rapid processing of visual information, whereas the *sustained system* handles slow-moving information, and the two systems are mutually inhibitory. In reading, the sustained system extracts detailed information during fixations, whilst the transient system extracts more general information from the periphery of vision, and integrates information from successive fixations. A major problem in reading is the persistence of information across fixations, which may result in the superimposition of images. In a series of studies of children with dyslexia, aged 8 to 15, Lovegrove demonstrated first that they showed a significantly smaller increase in visible persistence with increasing spatial frequency, which disappears when transient activity is reduced by the addition of a flicker field mask. A second approach showed some evidence for differences in contrast sensitivity to patterns, again abolished by flicker masking. Finally, a direct measure of transient system processing, based on flicker thresholds, differentiated well between the groups, and was supported by evidence from evoked potential studies. By contrast, there was little evidence for any deficit in the sustained system. Lovegrove goes on to investigate the role of the transient system in higher-order perceptual processing, using a technique known as metacontrast masking in which the target is presented briefly, followed at various intervals by a spatially adjacent mask. The mask delay which causes maximum disruption to target reading can be used to estimate the difference in speed between transient and sustained systems. Dyslexic subjects showed maximal disruption at shorter delay than the controls, from which Lovegrove infers that the dyslexic children's transient system was operating more slowly than normal.

The results obtained from these experiments are all consistent with the view that dyslexic children show a deficit in the transient system (but not the sustained system), and in a further test of the hypothesis two reading studies were undertaken: first, material was presented 'one word at a time', and, as hypothesised, this led to better reading by the dyslexics, based on the avoidance of the need for either eye movements or the integration of information. Second, blue light is thought to stimulate the transient channel relative to the sustained channel. Lovegrove cites experiments which suggest that use of blue light produces a normal time course of metacontrast in dyslexic children, and also that blue light leads to better general comprehension in dyslexic children than does white or red light. To conclude the chapter, Lovegrove links his results to known deficits in phonological coding, and suggests that both visual and phonological deficits may be attributable to a more generalised deficit in the processing of rapidly presented material in all sensory modalities, a suggestion reinforced by Stein in the following chapter.

In Chapter 5, John Stein re-examines the evidence for a visual deficit in dyslexia in terms of recent evidence for a transient system deficit. He argues that there is evidence that both visual and phonological deficits may be present in dyslexia, based on a more generalised abnormality of neurons in the central nervous system responsible for the processing of rapid signals. Stein's work has been primarily on ocular dominance, and he reviews studies which suggest that dyslexic children have unstable dominance, using the Dunlop test as a measure of binocular instability. In one study a cohort of children were followed for three years after school entry, and it was found that the rate at which dominance was established was a strong predictor of subsequent progress in reading. If dyslexic children suffer from unstable vergence, this should also be evident in a dot localisation task, where a second dot is displayed slightly to the left or right of the first dot for 200 ms, with the distance adjusted for each child to their 75% threshold. The results showed many more errors for dyslexic children, in a pattern similar to patients with right parietal lesions. In terms of reading errors, experimental work showed that this group consistently made more nonword errors in reading, and phonetic errors in spelling, even when their performance was compared with reading-age controls, and that these differences could be decreased by simply increasing the size of the print.

Stein argues that these results indicate that the visual deficits are a cause rather than an effect of the reading deficit and that both deficits may be ameliorated by the use of monocular occlusion or patching. Finally, Stein shows that in two distinct groups of children there is evidence for the presence of phonological deficits, as measured by the Bradley rhyming task, concurrently with the visual deficits. He interprets these results in terms of an impairment in temporal aspects of sensory and motor performance, and speculates that these are genetically based.

Chapter 6, by Fawcett and Nicolson, also reviews non-phonological skill deficits in dyslexic children, starting with the difficulties in rapid processing identified by several authors in this volume (Beech, Yap, Lovegrove and Stein), and describing a recent study in which they identified abnormalities even with a simple choice reaction task with non-phonological (pure tone) stimuli. Interestingly, however, speed of simple reaction was at normal levels. They then review the literature on motor skill, concluding that there are also difficulties with most motor skills, especially at young ages. In an attempt to provide a theoretical basis for analysis of this range of difficulties, they then broaden the scope of enquiry to consider theoretical analyses of the general processes of skill acquisition. On the basis of this analysis, the authors note that automaticity is a critical component of skilled behaviour, and put forward their 'Dyslexic Automaticity Deficit' (DAD) hypothesis as a potential explanatory construct in understanding the range of problems suffered by dyslexic children. There follows a description of three studies investigating the hypothesis undertaken by the authors. First, they describe a test of DAD using the motor skill of balance, a skill on which adolescent dyslexic children were thought to be unimpaired. Precisely as predicted by DAD, balance deficits were indeed found for dyslexic children. Most interestingly, these deficits were not apparent under normal conditions, but showed up only when the subjects were required to undertake a secondary task while balancing (or when blindfolded). The authors take this dissociation to indicate that the dyslexic children were impaired on balance, but could normally mask the deficit by 'conscious compensation' (concentrating hard on balancing), whereas non-dyslexic children are able to balance automatically, and are therefore little affected by secondary tasks.

Fawcett and Nicolson next describe two experiments designed to investigate further the nature of the hypothesised automatisation deficit, using a long-term training paradigm where matched groups of dyslexic and control children are given extensive training on a skill over several months, and the profile of the performance improvements is analysed to identify where, if at all, the learning shows abnormalities. In the first training study, which investigated acquisition of skill at a simple eye–hand coordination task involving navigation round a fixed circuit of a computer maze, the dyslexic children were considerably worse initially, and also after extended training, being not only slower but also much more error-prone; nonetheless the dyslexic children did show a normal rate of learning. The second study investigated the improvements with practice in speed of a two-choice reaction. Again, there were profound initial deficits (despite normal speed on a simple reaction to either of the two stimuli), and again the deficits persisted despite training. The authors conclude that, given the right circumstances, dyslexic children are able to learn at normal or near-normal rates, and may even acquire many of the characteristics of automatic performance, but that both initial and final performance will be characterised as more error-prone and more effortful than normal.

CHAPTER 4

Visual deficits in dyslexia: Evidence and implications

William Lovegrove

For some time it has been the view within the reading disability literature that reading disability is not attributable to visual deficits and that normal readers and dyslexics do not differ systematically in terms of visual processing (Benton, 1962; Vellutino, 1979a, b). Extensive work over the last ten years in a number of laboratories, however, has clearly demonstrated that the two groups do differ in terms of visual processing. This has been brought about partly by developments in theoretical vision which have been applied to reading thus providing a more meaningful theoretical context in which to consider reading disability and vision. Even though the more recent research has shown that many controls and dyslexics do differ in visual processing, the evidence on whether this relationship is causal is just emerging. Some of these data will be discussed here.

This chapter will review some of this research. In addition I will consider two possible implications of these data. First, I will consider whether there are any remedial implications which follow from it. Second, I will consider whether it may be indicative of a more general problem in dyslexia. The following section outlines one approach to vision which has been usefully applied to the study of dyslexia by a number of groups including our own.

SPATIAL FREQUENCY PROCESSING

One approach to vision research (Campbell, 1974; Graham, 1980) indicates that information is transmitted from the eye to the brain via a number of separate parallel pathways. The separate pathways are frequently referred to as channels. Each channel is specialised to process information about particular features of visual stimuli. The properties of channels often have been investigated using patterns composed of black and white bars with fuzzy edges. These patterns are usually called sine-wave gratings. Two properties of sine-wave gratings are important to the research outlined in this chapter.

Spatial frequency refers to the number of cycles (one dark plus one light bar) per degree of visual angle (c/deg) in a pattern. High spatial frequency patterns contain narrow bars and are believed to stimulate the channels which process detail. Low spatial frequency patterns contain very broad bars and stimulate channels which transmit information about general shape. Contrast refers to the difference between the maximum and minimum luminances of the grating. It is a measure of the ratio of the brightest to the darkest section of the pattern.

Research (Campbell, 1974; Graham, 1980) has identified a number of channels each sensitive to a narrow range of spatial frequencies (or stimulus widths) and orientations in cats, monkeys and humans. These are referred to as spatial frequency or size-sensitive channels.

Spatial frequency or size-sensitive channels are relevant to reading because when we read we process both general (low spatial frequency) and detailed (high spatial frequency) information in each fixation. We extract detailed information from an area approximately 5–6 letter spaces to the right of fixation. Beyond this we also extract visual information but only of a general nature such as word shape (Rayner, 1975). These two types of size information must in some way be combined across fixations.

Several studies have shown that these different channels transmit their information at different rates and respond differently to different rates of temporal change. Some channels are sensitive to very rapidly changing stimuli and others to stationary or slowly moving stimuli. In general, channels which are sensitive to low spatial frequencies are highly sensitive to rapid temporal change while channels sensitive to high spatial frequencies are insensitive to rapid temporal change. Evidence for this will be discussed in the next section. Such results have led to the proposal of two subsystems within the visual system. This division is believed to be important in combining the two types of size information involved in reading.

The sustained and transient subsystems

It has been shown that spatial frequency channels differ in their responses to changing stimuli. In a typical experiment subjects are shown sine-wave patterns flickering at various rates. Subjects are required to set contrast levels so that they just can see either flicker or pattern. When low spatial frequency gratings are moving quickly, we see flicker at lower contrasts than we see pattern but we experience the reverse at high spatial frequencies. Separate measures can be taken of our sensitivity to flicker and pattern with a range of different sized stimuli (spatial frequencies) flickering at different speeds. We can then plot sensitivity functions for pattern and flicker thresholds at a range of spatial frequencies. With large stimuli (low spatial frequencies) we are more sensitive to rapidly changing stimuli but with small stimuli (high spatial frequencies) we are more sensitive to stationary or slowly moving stimuli. The two functions obtained from such experiments are believed to measure two subsystems in the visual system, the transient and sustained subsystems. An extensive discussion of the properties of these systems and how they are identified can be found in Breitmeyer (1988). Breitmeyer also discusses the evidence indicating the physiological basis of these two systems. The properties of these two subsystems have been identified and are shown in Table 4.1.

It has been demonstrated physiologically (Singer and Bedworth, 1973) and psychophysically (Breitmeyer and Ganz, 1976) that the two systems may inhibit each other. In particular if the sustained system is responding when the transient system is stimulated, the transient system will terminate the sustained activity. An example of how this may occur is as follows. If we are fixating on the detail of an object and a stimulus moves into the periphery of our vision, the transient system is likely to inhibit or override the sustained system until we know what is in our peripheral vision. How this may have evolved is easier to imagine if we consider not a human reading but a rabbit eating and a predator appearing to the side. There would be survival value for the rabbit in having the transient system inhibit the sustained system until the level of threat could be determined.

Table 4.1 General properties of the sustained and transient subsystems

Sustained System	Transient System
Less sensitive to contrast	Highly sensitive to contrast
Most sensitive to high spatial frequencies	Most sensitive to low spatial frequencies
Most sensitive to low temporal frequencies	Most sensitive to high temporal frequencies
Slow transmission times	Fast transmission times
Responds throughout stimulus presentation	Responds at stimulus onset and offset
Predominates in central vision	Predominates in peripheral vision
The sustained system may inhibit the transient system	The transient system may inhibit the sustained system

The transient system is predominantly a flicker or motion detecting system transmitting information about stimulus change and general shape. The spatial information it transmits is coarse and thus well suited for transmitting peripheral information in reading. The sustained system is predominantly a detailed pattern detecting system transmitting information about stationary stimuli. In reading the sustained system should be most important in extracting detailed information during fixations and the transient system in extracting general information from the periphery. The transient system has also been implicated in the important task of integrating information from successive fixations. These two subsystems and the interactions between them may serve a number of functions essential to the reading process. Below we shall see that the two systems also interact in important ways.

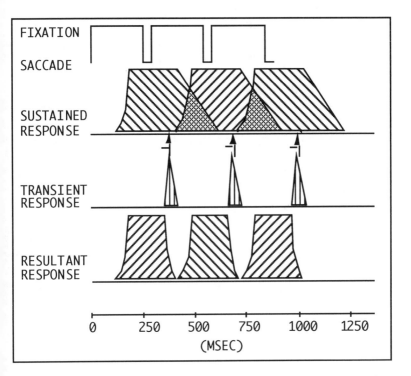

Figure 4.1 A hypothetical response sequence of sustained and transient channels during 3 250 ms fixation intervals separated by 25 ms saccades (top panel). Panel 2 illustrates persistence of sustained channels acting as a forward mask from preceding to succeeding fixation intervals. Panel 3 shows the activation of transient channels shortly after each saccade which exerts inhibition (arrows with minus signs) on the trailing, persisting sustained activity generated in prior fixation intervals. Panel 4 shows the resultant sustained channel response after the effects of the transient-on-sustained inhibition have been taken into account (Adapted from B. G. Breitmeyer, Unmasking visual masking: A look at the 'Why' behind the veil of the 'How' *Psychological Review*, 1980, *82*, 52–69. Copyright 1980 by the American Psychological Association. Permission to reprint granted.)

Sustained and transient subsystems and reading

When reading, the eyes move through a series of rapid eye movements called saccades. These are separated by fixation intervals when the eyes are stationary. Saccadic eye movements are generally in the direction of reading, that is, from left to right when reading English. Sometimes the eyes also move from right to left in what are called regressive eye movements or regressions. The average fixation duration is approximately 200–250 ms for normal readers and it is during these stationary periods that information from the printed page is seen. The average saccade length is 6–8 characters, or about 2 degrees of visual angle (Rayner and McConkie, 1976). Saccadic eye movements function to bring unidentified regions of text into foveal vision for detailed analysis during fixations. Foveal vision is the area of high acuity in the centre of vision extending approximately 2 degrees (6–8 letters) around the fixation point on a line of text. Beyond the fovea acuity drops off rather dramatically.

The role of transient and sustained subsystems in reading has been considered by Breitmeyer (Breitmeyer, 1980; 1983; 1988; Breitmeyer and Ganz, 1976). Figure 4.1 represents the hypothesised activity in the transient and sustained channels over a sequence of three fixations of 250 ms duration separated by two saccades of 25 ms duration each.

The sustained channel response occurs during fixations and may last for several hundred milliseconds. This response provides details of what the eye is seeing. The transient channel response is initiated by eye movements and lasts for much shorter durations. Consequently, both systems are involved in reading. The duration of the sustained response may outlast the physical duration of the stimulus. This is a form of visible persistence produced by activating sustained channels. Its duration increases with increasing spatial frequency (Bowling, Lovegrove and Mapperson, 1979; Meyer and Maguire, 1977) and may last longer than a saccade.

If sustained activity (as shown in Figure 4.1, second panel down) generated in a preceding fixation persists into the succeeding one, it may interfere with processing there. In this case, what may happen when reading a line of print requiring one, two or three fixations is illustrated in Figure 4.2 (adapted from Hochberg, 1978).

Consequently, it is evident that for tasks such as reading, persistence across saccades presents a problem as it may lead to superimposition of successive inputs. Breitmeyer proposes that the problem posed by visible persistence is solved by rapid saccades as shown in the bottom two panels of Figure 4.1. Saccades not only change visual fixations, they also activate short latency transient channels (panel 3) which are very sensitive to stimulus movement. This, in turn, inhibits the sustained activity which would persist from a preceding fixation and interfere with the succeeding one (Breitmeyer and Ganz, 1976; Matin, 1974). The result is a series of clear, unmasked and temporally segregated frames of sustained activity, each one representing the pattern information contained in a single fixation as shown in panel 4 of Figure 4.1.

NORMAL VI**N**O**R**MA**I**L SV **N**O**R**M**A**O**I**L**A**S**I**E**I**CONO**L**A**S**I **I**CONOCLASTIC	(THREE FIXATIONS)
NORMAL VISION N**S**O**R**M**A**O**O**N**I**O**S**I**A**G**N**I **I**S ICONOCLASTIC	(TWO FIXATIONS)
NORMAL VISION IS ICONOCLASTIC	(ONE FIXATION)

Figure 4.2 The perceptual masking effects of temporal integration of persisting sustained activity from preceding fixation intervals with sustained activity generated in succeeding ones when the reading of a printed sentence requires one, two or three fixations. Here, as in panel 2 of Figure 4.1, the effects of transient-on-sustained inhibition have not been taken into account. (Adapted from B. G. Breitmeyer, Unmasking visual masking: A look at the 'Why' behind the veil of the 'How' *Psychological Review*, 1980, *82*, 52–69. Copyright 1980 by the American Psychological Association. Permission to reprint granted.)

In these terms, clear vision on each fixation results from interactions between the sustained and transient channels. Consequently, the nature of transient–sustained channel interaction seems to be important in facilitating normal reading. Any problem in either the transient or the sustained system or in the way they interact may have harmful consequences for reading.

Transient and sustained processing in dyslexics and controls

The possibility of a visual deficit in dyslexics has recently been investigated within the theoretical framework of spatial frequency analysis. The following is not a complete review of all recent research but a summary of the research carried out in a few laboratories including ours. Subjects in the studies by Lovegrove and colleagues have normally been chosen to have at least normal intelligence and a reading accuracy lag of at least two years on the Neale Analysis of Reading Ability (1966). Much of this research has been directed at the functioning of the transient and sustained systems in normal and specifically disabled readers.

Low-level visual processing in dyslexics and controls

Visible persistence is one measure of temporal processing in spatial frequency channels and refers to the continued perception of a stimulus after it has been physically removed. The top panel in Figure 4.1 demonstrates such persistence. This is assumed to reflect ongoing neural activity initiated by the stimulus presentation. In adults, duration of visible persistence increases with increasing spatial frequency (Bowling *et al.*, 1979; Meyer and Maguire, 1977). Several studies have compared dyslexics and controls on measures of visible persistence. It has been shown that dyslexics aged from 8 to 15 years have a significantly smaller increase in persistence duration with increasing spatial frequency than do controls (Badcock and Lovegrove, 1981; Lovegrove, Heddle and Slaghuis, 1980; Slaghuis and Lovegrove, 1985).

When visible persistence is measured in both groups under conditions which reduce transient system activity (using a uniform field flicker mask), persistence differences between the groups essentially disappear (Slaghuis and Lovegrove, 1984). This finding suggests that dyslexics may differ from controls mainly in the functioning of their transient systems.

The two groups have also been compared on a task which measures the minimum contrast required to see a pattern. Contrast sensitivity (the reciprocal of the minimum contrast required for detection), plotted as a function of spatial frequency, is referred to as the contrast sensitivity function (CSF). Pattern CSFs have been measured in at least five separate samples of dyslexics and control readers with ages ranging from 8 years to 14 years. It has generally been shown that dyslexics are less sensitive than controls at low (1.0–4 c/deg) spatial frequencies (Lovegrove *et al.*, 1980; Lovegrove *et al.*, 1982; Martin and Lovegrove, 1984). In some studies the two groups do not differ in contrast sensitivity at higher (12–16 c/deg) spatial frequencies (Lovegrove *et al.*, 1980) and in others dyslexics are slightly more sensitive than controls in that range (Lovegrove *et al.*, 1982; Martin and Lovegrove, 1984). At high luminances dyslexics have been found to be less sensitive at high spatial frequencies than controls. Once again attenuation of the transient system by uniform-field masking influenced the dyslexics less than controls (Martin and Lovegrove, 1988) thus further supporting the notion of a difference between the groups in the transient system.

A third approach has been to measure transient system functioning more directly than did the previous two measures. It has been argued that flicker thresholds are primarily mediated by the transient system. Consequently, flicker thresholds under a range of conditions have been measured in dyslexics and controls. In these experiments subjects are shown a sine-wave grating counterphasing, i.e., moving from right to left and back the distance of one cycle at whatever speed the experimenter chooses. Subjects are required to detect the presence of the flicker. In a number of experiments dyslexics have been shown to be less sensitive than controls to counterphase flicker (Brannan and Williams, 1988; Martin and Lovegrove, 1987; 1988). The differences between the groups sometimes become larger as the temporal frequency increases (Martin and Lovegrove, 1987; 1988) and sometimes do not (Brannan and Williams, 1988). What happens depends on the spatial make-up of the stimuli. This is a direct measure of transient system processing and distinguishes very well between individuals in the two groups (Martin and Lovegrove, 1987).

Additional support for differences between the groups in terms of spatial frequency processing comes from recent visual evoked potential studies (Livingstone *et al.*, 1991; May *et al.*, 1991; May, Dunlap and Lovegrove, 1991). In the study by May *et al.* subjects were presented with sine-wave gratings ranging in spatial frequency from 0.5 to 8.0 cycles per degree flickering at a rate of two Hertz (Hz). Stimulus duration was 200 ms. This allowed analysis of two components of the VEP elicited by both stimulus onset and by stimulus offset. The major findings indicated that poor readers had significantly lower amplitudes and significantly shorter latencies for components produced by stimulus offsets when low spatial frequency stimuli were used.

Factor analyses of latency scores from this study revealed two factors for both the low and high spatial frequency stimuli (May, Dunlap and Lovegrove, 1992). With the low spatial frequency stimulus, Factor II was associated with the latencies on the first onset component and Factor I with the latencies of all components. These scores were subject to a discriminant analysis which showed that good and poor readers were well differentiated by the factor scores on the low spatial frequency but not the high spatial frequency factor. This is consistent with a problem in the transient system. Further visual-evoked potential data supporting this conclusion but using different conditions have been reported (Livingstone *et al.*, 1991).

Lovegrove and associates have also conducted a series of experiments comparing sustained system processing in controls and dyslexics (see Lovegrove *et al.*, 1986). Using similar procedures, equipment and subjects as the experiments outlined above, this series of experiments has failed to show any significant differences between the two groups. These data suggest that either there are no differences between the groups in the functioning of their sustained systems or that such differences are smaller than the transient differences demonstrated.

In summary, four converging lines of evidence suggest a transient deficit in dyslexics. The differences between the groups are quite large on some measures and discriminate well between individuals in the different groups with approximately 75% of dyslexics showing reduced transient system sensitivity (Slaghuis and Lovegrove, 1985). At the same time evidence to date suggests that the two groups do not differ in sustained system functioning.

Higher-level perceptual processes and dyslexia

It is known that the transient and sustained systems may be involved in perceptual processes at a higher level than those discussed above (Breitmeyer and Ganz, 1976; Weisstein, Ozog and Szoc, 1975). Williams and colleagues have recently investigated how a transient deficit may manifest itself in a range of higher-level perceptual processes. It should be noted that Williams and colleagues have on average worked with younger subjects than Lovegrove and colleagues and have chosen subjects with reading lags of about 18 months. Their general conclusion (Williams and LeCluyse, 1990) is that dyslexics manifest difficulties on a large number of perceptual tasks, most of which are believed to involve the transient system.

In an important study, Williams, Molinet and LeCluyse (1989) plotted the time course of transient–sustained interactions. A standard way of measuring the temporal properties of transient–sustained interactions is to use a metacontrast masking paradigm (Breitmeyer and Ganz, 1976). In metacontrast masking a target is briefly presented followed at various delays by a spatially adjacent masking stimulus. The experiment measures the effect of the mask on the visibility of the target. The target is affected by both the temporal and spatial relationship between the mask and the target. It is normally found that the visibility of the target first decreases and then increases as the pattern mask follows it by longer and longer delays. Breitmeyer and Weisstein have argued that metacontrast masking is due to the inhibition of the sustained response to the target by the transient response to the mask. This happens in much the same way sustained persistence is terminated by transient activity during reading as is shown in Figure 4.2.

Maximal masking occurs when the transient response to the mask and the sustained response to the target overlap most in time in the visual system. This occurs in metacontrast when the mask follows the target by a certain interval. The point of maximal masking, then, provides an index of the relative processing rates of the target sustained response and the mask transient response. If the difference in rate of transmission is small, the dip in the masking function occurs after a short delay and vice versa. The magnitude of masking provides an index of the strength of transient-on-sustained inhibition. Additionally metacontrast is normally stronger in peripheral than in central viewing presumably because of the preponderance of transient pathways in peripheral vision. It should be noted that this is the same mechanism proposed to be involved in saccadic suppression (the suppression of sustained activity during eye movements) as discussed earlier in relation to Figures 4.1 and 4.2.

In an experiment using line targets, Williams, Molinet and LeCluyse (1989) showed that maximal masking occurred at a shorter delay in dyslexics than in controls. This result is direct evidence that dyslexics have a slower transient system or at least a smaller difference between the rates of processing for their transient and sustained systems than controls. They also found that in peripheral vision dyslexics experienced almost no metacontrast masking, which further supports this position. The magnitude of masking was also less in central vision showing that the transient inhibition was also weaker. Further evidence supporting timing differences between the transient and sustained systems in controls and dyslexics has been provided in another metacontrast experiment where subjects had to identify a target letter. The mask was also letters but could combine with the target to form a word or a nonword (Williams, Brannan and Bologna, 1988). Both of these studies provide clear evidence of temporal differences between the two groups contributing to high-level perceptual problems.

In summary, there is now a large number of studies which have investigated higher-level perceptual processing in good and poor readers. The results from this wide range of measures confirm the finding of a transient deficit in dyslexics. They also suggest that there may be other deficits (visual and higher level) but the precise nature of these is not yet clear.

At least three questions emerge from the demonstration that dyslexics and controls do differ in at least one aspect of visual processing. The first concerns the possible explanations for the conflicting findings reported in the literature. The second addresses the important applied issue of whether any 'visual' manipulations are likely to assist dyslexic children to read. The third question concerns the possible relationship between visual deficits and other documented deficits experienced by dyslexics. These will be discussed in turn.

WHAT ABOUT THE CONFUSION IN THE LITERATURE?

Over the years a substantial number of studies have reported differences in visual processing between good and poor readers. Several researchers (Blackwell, Mcintyre and Murray, 1983; Di Lollo, Hanson and Mcintyre, 1983; Hoien, 1980; Lovegrove and Brown, 1978; Stanley and Hall, 1973) have shown that masking occurs over longer durations in dyslexics than in controls. Mason, Pilkington and Brandau (1981) have shown dyslexics to have difficulties with order rather than item information. Hyvarinen and Laurinen (1980) have measured spatial and temporal processing across spatial frequencies. They generally found that disabled readers were less sensitive than controls, without specifying whether this difference was greater at certain spatial frequencies.

The difficulty in making sense of this literature, however, is that for almost every study showing differences between the two groups another study may be cited failing to show differences. For example, Arnett and di Lollo (1979), Fisher and Frankfurter (1977), Morrison, Giordani and Nagy (1977) and Manis and Morrison (1982) have all conducted studies with short-duration stimuli without finding any significant differences between groups. Howell, Smith and Stanley (1981) and Smith, Early and Grogan (1986) failed to show spatial-frequency specific differences in visible persistence between the two groups.

An obvious question is whether it is possible to reconcile these different sets of results in terms of the argument presented here. In the context of this chapter it may be suggested that many of the studies which have failed to show differences between dyslexics and normal readers in visual processing may have measured sustained processing and those which have shown differences have measured either transient system processing or transient–sustained interactions. Support for this position has recently been provided by Meca (1985), who has conducted a meta-analysis on a large number of studies investigating vision and reading. He plotted effect size as a function of spatial frequency. As would be expected if dyslexics had a transient system problem but not a sustained system problem, effect size was greatest at low spatial frequencies and decreased with increasing spatial frequency (Meca, 1985).

While this is almost certainly oversimplistic it does allow us to make predictions about what should be found on a range of different tasks depending on whether or not transient or sustained processing is being measured. A recent study (Solman and May, 1990) has investigated spatial localisation in dyslexic and normal readers within this context. They predicted not only conditions where dyslexics should be worse than controls but also where dyslexics would perform at least as well or even better than controls. They found that when the targets were close to the fixation points dyslexics performed slightly better than controls. This pattern reversed as the targets moved more into peripheral vision (and were presumably processed more by the transient system). It may be stated, therefore, that while there is a large amount of data consistent with the argument presented here there are also substantial data inconsistent with it. The consistent data are, generally, more recent and have formed part of one of a small number of systematic programmes of research. If the argument presented here is valid, it is possible to make clear predictions about the types of visual tasks on which dyslexics should do worse and/or better than controls.

It is important to note in this context that recent research has not simply demonstrated dyslexics performing more poorly than controls on all measures of visual processing. Dyslexics have been shown to perform at least as well as or even better than controls on some tasks, e.g., high spatial frequency sensitivity, visual acuity and the oblique effect (Lovegrove *et al.*, 1986). Generally, this is thought to be the case on tasks measuring sustained system functioning. Further experimentation will determine whether or not this is so.

REMEDIAL IMPLICATIONS

Two approaches to this question have so far been investigated. The first has manipulated the nature of visual presentation during reading and the second has attempted to modify the relative balance of the transient and sustained subsystems.

The one word at a time advantage

Lovegrove and colleagues attempted to predict from Breitmeyer's theory the effect that different types of spatial context may have on reading accuracy in dyslexics and controls. In terms of Breitmeyer's theory outlined earlier a transient deficit should lead to more errors for dyslexics when reading continuous text than when reading isolated words. This is because reading continuous text requires integration of peripheral information from one fixation with central information on the next. This has been tested by varying the mode of visual presentation (Hill and Lovegrove, 1992; Lovegrove and MacFarlane, 1990). Three conditions of visual presentation on a computer monitor were used while holding the semantic context constant. This was done by presenting stories in three different ways. In the first condition one word at a time was presented in the middle of the screen. Thus the subjects never had to move their eyes and never had information presented to the right of fixation. In the second condition one word was presented at a time but its position was moved across the screen so that each successive word appeared to the right of the previous word. Once a word was presented, it remained on the screen so that at the end of the line, a whole line of print was present. Here the subjects were required to move their eyes across the screen but still were never presented with information to the right of fixation. The final condition was a whole line presentation which most closely approximated normal reading. Rate of word presentation was held constant across the three conditions.

The results (Hill and Lovegrove, 1992; Lovegrove and MacFarlane, 1990) showed normal readers were most accurate in the whole line condition and made more errors in the two one word at time conditions. The reverse was true for the dyslexics. They read significantly more accurately in both one-word conditions than the whole-line condition. We refer to this as the 'one word at a time advantage'.

There were no differences for the dyslexics between the two one word at a time conditions. This suggests that they did not experience any additional problems when required to move their eyes but did experience difficulties when they had to integrate print to the right of fixation with centrally presented text. It is worth commenting that this is quite a large effect and has found with nearly all dyslexics we have tested (about 30). The mode of presentation of written material which maximised reading accuracy in controls, therefore, produced the most errors in dyslexics. Although the exact reason for this effect is to be determined, the finding may have remedial implications. These are currently being further investigated.

The effects of wavelength filtering

If a deficient transient system does play a role in reading disabilities, any manipulation which enhances transient system functioning relative to sustained system functioning may assist with reading. Some data from vision research have provided a means by which to consider this possibility.

Recent psychophysical and physiological data indicate that colour or wavelength differentially affect the response characteristics of transient and sustained processing channels, and that wavelength can affect the relative contributions of transient and sustained channels to the processing of a stimulus. Physiological observations of the primate visual system indicate that there are differences in the colour selectivity of these systems (Livingstone and Hubel, 1987), and that a steady red background light attenuates the response of transient channels (Dreher, Fukuda and Rodieck, 1976; Kruger, 1977; Schiller and Malpeli, 1978). A recent investigation by Breitmeyer and Williams (1990) provides evidence that variations in wavelength produce similar effects in the human visual system. They found that the magnitude of both metacontrast and stroboscopic motion was decreased when red as compared with equiluminant green or white backgrounds were used. According to transient–sustained theories of metacontrast and stroboscopic motion, these results indicate that the activity of transient channels is attenuated by red backgrounds. Williams *et al.* (1991), using a metacontrast paradigm, additionally found that the rate of processing in transient channels increases as wavelength decreases (i.e., towards the blue end of the spectrum), and that red light enhances the activity of sustained channels.

These results indicate that wavelength would provide a means of modifying the relative functioning of the transient and sustained systems.

Williams, LeCluyse and Bologna (1990) used a metacontrast paradigm to obtain direct measures of the effects of colour on temporal visual processing in normal and disabled readers. They found that the metacontrast functions obtained with dyslexics in blue light were very similar to those obtained with controls in white light in terms of both the magnitude of masking and the stimulus-onset asynchrony at which maximum masking occurred. In other words, the function produced by the blue mask in dyslexics is similar in time course to the function produced by the white mask in normal readers. This finding suggests that blue light produces a normal time course of processing in disabled readers, and is consistent with the contention that blue light may enhance the processing rate in transient channels.

Given the systematic effects of colour on the perceptual

performance of the reading disabled, and the fact that this manipulation can render their performance comparable to that of normal readers, Williams *et al.,* (1990) investigated the effects of colour on actual reading performance. They did this by measuring reading comprehension in three conditions similar to those used by Lovegrove and MacFarlane (1990) and outlined in the previous section. Their results showed that dyslexics generally comprehended text better when it was presented in blue than in white or red light. While Williams and colleagues have yet to determine the long-term effects of wavelength on reading, these results on comprehension are interesting and again suggest a possible remedial direction.

Thus there is preliminary work on two remedial approaches derived from our knowledge of a specific visual deficit in dyslexia. While much work has yet to be done, the results to date are promising and are currently being pursued further.

POSSIBLE RELATIONSHIP TO OTHER PROBLEMS MANIFEST IN DYSLEXIA?

A final implication for consideration resulting from the work on vision and dyslexia concerns any possible relationship between the visual deficits described here and other known deficits in dyslexia. There is extensive evidence that dyslexics perform worse than controls in a number of other areas, especially in aspects of phonological awareness and working memory. It becomes important to ask what, if any, is the relation between the transient system deficits and these other processing areas.

This issue was considered in a recent study of approximately 60 dyslexics and 60 controls (Lovegrove *et al.*, 1988). They took measures of transient system processing, phonological awareness, phonological recoding and working memory in each child. These measures were subjected to a factor analysis which showed that phonological recoding as measured by nonsense word ability loaded on the same factor as the measures of transient processing used. This shows some relation between the two processing areas but, of course, does not reveal the precise nature of that relationship.

Until this relationship is further clarified it is premature to reject the possibility of a link between visual and phonological processes in reading. The measures of working memory used did not load on the same factor as did the transient system measures and the phonological recoding measures. This study thus provides some preliminary evidence of a link between phonological recoding and visual processing in dyslexics but the exact nature of this relation is still to be determined.

It is possible that some of these different deficits are related by virtue of the fact that some dyslexics have a problem in processing rapidly presented stimuli in all sensory modalities. Tallal (1980), for example, has shown that dyslexics have temporal problems in audition which may be auditory analogues of the visual transient system deficits we have studied. This possibility has recently been speculated on by Livingstone *et al.* (1991), who noted that the auditory and somatosensory systems may also be subdivided into fast and slow components like the visual system. They then speculated that problems in each fast system may occur in dyslexics. If this were so, a rapid temporal processing deficit in dyslexics may contribute to their problems in phonological awareness. Even though this possibility has not yet been directly investigated, it is an exciting prospect which may help to integrate a large amount of apparently discrepant data. Such a framework linking visual processing, phonological awareness and phonological awareness makes some intuitive sense. Any more direct link is hard to foresee.

CONCLUSIONS

The data reported in the last ten years show that many dyslexics have a particular visual deficit. It has also been shown that it is unlikely that the transient deficit results from being unable to read (Lovegrove *et al.*, 1986) although it is not yet known how it may contribute to reading difficulties. This problem appears to be present in a large percentage of disabled readers and not just for a subgroup frequently referred to as visuo-spatial dyslexics. There is still a lot of work to be done before knowing how this processing difficulty relates to other difficulties but one interesting possibility has been outlined. The results with different modes of visual presentation and with the effects of wavelength on reading in dyslexics and controls will be further investigated in our laboratory and are encouraging.

REFERENCES

Arnett, J.L. and Di Lollo, V. (1979). Visual information processing in relation to age and reading ability. *Journal of Experimental Child Psychology, 27*, 143–152.

Badcock, D.R. and Lovegrove, W. (1981). The effect of contrast, stimulus duration and spatial frequency on visible persistence in normal and specifically disabled readers. *Journal of Experimental Psychology: Human perception and performance, 7*, 495–505.

Benton, A.L. (1962). Dyslexia in relation to form perception and directional sense. In J. Money (Ed.), *Reading Disability: Progress and research needs in dyslexia* (pp. 81–102). Baltimore: Johns Hopkins Press.

Blackwell, S., McIntyre, D. and Murray, M. (1983). Information processing from brief visual displays by learning disabled boys. *Child Development, 54*, 927–940.

Bowling, A., Lovegrove W. and Mapperson, B. (1979). The effect of spatial frequency and contrast on visible persistence. *Perception, 8*, 529–539.

Bradley, L. and Bryant, P. (1983). Categorising sounds and learning to read – a causal connection. *Nature, 301*, 419–421.

Brannan, J. and Williams, M. (1988). The effects of age and reading ability on flicker threshold. *Clinical Visual Sciences, 3*, 137–142.

Breitmeyer, B.G. (1980). Unmasking visual masking: A look at the 'why' behind the veil of 'how'. *Psychological Review, 87*, 52–69.

Breitmeyer, B.G. (1983). Sensory masking, persistence and enhancement in visual exploration and reading. In K. Rayner (Ed.), *Eye Movements in Reading: Perceptual and language processes.* New York: Academic Press.

Breitmeyer, B.G. (1988). Reality and relevance of sustained and transient channels in reading and reading disability. *Paper presented to the 24th International Congress of Psychology*, Sydney.

Breitmeyer, B.G. and Ganz, L. (1976). Implications of sustained and transient channels for theories of visual pattern making, saccadic suppression and information processing. *Psychological Review, 83*, 1–36.

Breitmeyer, B.G. and Williams, M.C. (1990). Effects of isoluminant background colour on metacontrast and stroboscopic motion: Interactions between sustained (P) and transient (M) channels. *Vision Research, 30,* 1069–1075.

Campbell, F.W. (1974). The transmission of spatial information through the visual system. In F.O. Schmidt and F.S. Worden (Eds.), *The Neurosciences Third Study Program*, (pp. 95–103). Cambridge, MA: The MIT Press.

Di Lollo, V., Hanson D. and McIntyre, J. (1983). Initial stages of visual information processing in dyslexia. *Journal of Experimental Psychology: Human perception and performance, 9,* 923–935.

Dreher, B., Fukuda, Y. and Rodieck, R. (1976). Identification, classification and anatomical segregation of cells with X like and Y like properties in the lateral geniculate nucleus of old world primates. *Journal of Physiology, 258,* 433–452.

Fisher, D.F. and Frankfurter, A. (1977). Normal and disabled readers can locate and identify letters: Where's the perceptual deficit? *Journal of Reading Behaviour, 10,* 31–43.

Galaburda, A., Drislane, F. and Livingstone, M. (1991). Anatomical evidence for a magnocellular defect in developmental dyslexia. *Proceedings of the New York Academy of Sciences, 88.*

Graham, N. (1980). Spatial frequency channels in human vision. Detecting edges without edges detectors. In C.S. Harris (Ed.), *Visual Coding and Adaptability* (pp. 215–262). Hillsdale, NJ: Lawrence Erlbaum.

Hill, R and Lovegrove, W. (1992). One word at a time: A solution to the visual deficit in SRD's? In S.F. Wright and R. Groner, (Eds.), *Facets of Dyslexia and its Remediation* (pp. 65–77). Amsterdam: Elsevier.

Hochberg, J. E. (1978). *Perception.* Englewood Cliffs, NJ: Prentice-Hall.

Hoien, T. (1980). The relationship between iconic persistence and reading disabilities. In Y. Zotterman (Ed.), *Dyslexia: Neuronal, cognitive and linguistic aspects* (pp. 93–107). Oxford: Pergamon Press.

Howell, E.R., Smith, G.A. and Stanley, G. (1981). Reading disability and visual spatial frequency specific effects. *Australian Journal of Psychology, 33,* 97–102.

Hyvarinen, L. and Laurinen, P. (1980). Ophthalmological findings and contrast sensitivity in children with reading difficulties. In Y. Zotterman (Ed.), *Dyslexia: Neural, cognitive and linguistic aspects* (pp. 117–119). Oxford: Pergamon Press.

Livingstone, M. and Hubel, D. (1987). Psychophysical evidence for separate channels for the perception of form, color, movement and depth. *Journal of Neuroscience, 7,* 3416–3468.

Livingstone, M., Rosen, G.D., Drislane, F. and Galaburda, A. (1991). Physiological evidence for a magnocellular defect in developmental dyslexia. *Proceedings of the New York Academy of Sciences, 88,* 7943–

7947.

Lovegrove, W.J., Bowling, A., Badcock, D. and Blackwood, M. (1980). Specific reading disability: Differences in contrast sensitivity as a function of spatial frequency. *Science, 210*, 439–440.

Lovegrove, W.J. and Brown, C. (1978). Development of information processing in normal and disabled readers. *Perceptual and Motor Skills, 46*, 1047–1054.

Lovegrove, W., Heddle, M. and Slaghuis, W. (1980). Reading disability: Spatial frequency specific deficits in visual information store. *Neuropsychologia, 18*, 111–115.

Lovegrove W. and MacFarlane T. (1990). *How Can We Help SRDs in Learning to Read?* Unpublished honours thesis. University of Wollongong.

Lovegrove, W., Martin, F., Bowling, A., Badcock, D. and Paxton, S. (1982). Contrast sensitivity functions and specific reading disability. *Neuropsychologia, 20*, 309–315.

Lovegrove, W., Martin, F. and Slaghuis, W. (1986). A theoretical and experimental case for a residual deficit in specific reading disability. *Cognitive Neuropsychology, 3*, 225–267.

Lovegrove, W., McNicol, D., Martin, F., Mackenzie, B. and Pepper, K. (1988). Phonological recoding, memory processing and memory deficits in specific reading disability. In D. Vickers and P. Smith (Eds.), *Human Information Processing: Measures, mechanisms and models* (pp. 65–82). North-Holland: Amsterdam.

Manis, F.R. and Morrison, F.J. (1982). Processing of identity and position information in normal and disabled readers. *Journal of Experimental Child Psychology, 33*, 74–86.

Martin, F. and Lovegrove, W. (1984). The effects of field size and luminance on contrast sensitivity differences between specifically reading disabled and normal children. *Neuropsychologia, 22*, 73–77.

Martin, F. and Lovegrove, W. (1987). Flicker contrast sensitivity in normal and specifically-disabled readers. *Perception, 16*, 215–221.

Martin, F. and Lovegrove, W. (1988). Uniform and field flicker in control and specifically-disabled readers. *Perception, 17*, 203–214.

Mason, M., Pilkington, C. and Brandau, R. (1981). From print to sound: Reading ability and order information. *Journal of Experimental Psychology: Human Perception and Performance, 7*, 580–591.

Matin, E. (1974). Saccadic suppression: A review and an analysis. *Psychological Bulletin, 81*, 899–915.

May, J., Dunlap, W. and Lovegrove, W. (1991). Factor scores derived from visual evoked potentials differentiate good and poor readers. *Clinical Vision Sciences, 7*, 67-70.

May, J., Lovegrove, W., Martin, F. and Nelson, W. (1991). Pattern–elicited visual evoked potentials in good and poor readers. *Clinical Vision*

Sciences, 2, 131–136.

Meca, J. (1985). La hipotesis del deficit perceptivo del retraso especifico en lectura : un estudio meta–analitico. *Anales de Psicologia, 2,* 75–91.

Meyer, G.E. and Maguire, W.M. (1977). Spatial frequency and the mediation of short–term visual storage. *Science, 198,* 524–525.

Morrison, F., Giordani, B. and Nagy, J. (1977). Reading disability: An information processing analysis. *Science, 196,* 77–79.

Rayner, K. (1975). The perceptual span and peripheral cues in reading. *Cognitive Psychology, 7,* 65–81.

Rayner, K. and McConkie, G.W. (1976). What guides a reader's eye movements? *Vision Research, 16,* 829–837.

Schiller, P. and Malpeli, J. (1978). Functional specificity of lateral geniculate nucleus laminae of the rhesus monkey. *Journal of Neurophysiology, 41,* 788–797.

Singer, W. and Bedworth, N. (1973). Inhibitory interaction between X and Y units in the cat lateral geniculate nucleus. *Brain Research, 49,* 291–307.

Slaghuis, W. and Lovegrove, W.J. (1984). Flicker masking of spatial frequency dependent visible persistence and specific reading disability. *Perception, 13,* 527–534.

Slaghuis, W. and Lovegrove, W.J. (1985). Spatial-frequency mediated visible persistence and specific reading disability. *Brain and Cognition, 4,* 219–240.

Solman, R. and May, J. (1990). Spatial localisation discrepancies: A visual deficit in reading. *American Journal of Psychology, 103,* 243–263.

Smith, A., Early, F. and Grogan, S. (1986). Flicker masking and developmental dyslexia. *Perception, 15,* 473–482.

Stanley, G. and Hall, R. (1973). Short-term visual information processing in dyslexics. *Child Development, 44,* 841–844.

Tallal, P. (1980). Auditory temporal perception, phonics and reading disabilities in children. *Brain and Language, 9,* 182–198.

Vellutino, F.R. (1979a). The validity of perceptual deficit explanations of reading disability: A reply to Fletcher and Satz. *Journal of Learning Disabilities, 12,* 160–167.

Vellutino, F.R. (1979b). *Dyslexia: Theory and research.* London: MIT Press.

Weisstein, N., Ozoz, G. and Szoc, R. (1975). A comparison and elaboration of two models of metacontrast. *Psychological Review, 82,* 325–342.

Williams, M., Brannan, J. and Bologna, N. (1988). Perceptual consequences of a transient subsystem visual deficit in the reading disabled. *Paper presented to the 24th International Congress of Psychology,* Sydney.

Williams, M., Breitmeyer, B., Lovegrove, W. and Gutierrez, C. (1991). Metacontrast with masks varying in spatial frequency and wavelength. *Vision Research, 31,* 2017–2023.

Williams, M. and LeCluyse, K. (1990). Perceptual consequences of a temporal processing deficit in reading disabled children. *Journal of the American Optometry Association*, *61*, 111–121.

Williams, M.C., LeCluyse, K. and Bologna, N. (1990). Masking by light as a measure of visual integration time in normal and disabled readers. *Clinical Vision Sciences*, *5*, 335-343.

Williams, M., Molinet, K. and LeCluyse, K. (1989). Visual masking as a measure of temporal processing in normal and disabled readers. *Clinical Vision Sciences*, *4*, 137–144.

Williams, M.C., Weisstein, N., Rockfaucheux,A. and LeCluyse, K. (1990). Short-wavelength (blue) text improves reading comprehension in reading-disabled children *Bulletin of the Psychonomic Society*, *28*, 495.

CHAPTER 5

A visual defect in dyslexics?

J.F. Stein

Until 20 years ago children's reading difficulties were generally attributed to a defect in visual processing. Morgan used the term word blindness and Orton strephosymbolia (twisted symbols) to emphasise this view of their causation. More recently however the idea that visual perceptual problems have much to do with children's reading problems has given way to the view that defective development of phonological skills is more important. The evidence is now overwhelming that phonological ability is a strong determinant of reading progress, and that dyslexic children often have deficient skills in this area (Bradley and Bryant, 1983; Liberman et al., 1977; see also the chapters by Rack and Beech in this volume). Although this finding does not exclude a role for visual processing in reading development, other research seemed to indicate that there is no correlation at all between children's visual skills and their reading ability (Vellutino, 1987).

In the last few years however it has become clear that the visual system cannot be ignored when investigating reading difficulties. In this chapter I shall show that visual skills do in fact correlate remarkably well with reading performance, and that many children with reading problems have unstable visual perceptions which are probably caused by unstable visuomotor control. This leads them to experience visual confusions, hence they make characteristic 'visual' reading errors. Unstable visuomotor control may be a consequence of abnormality of the magnocellular, transient, component of the visual processing system. Usually the visual abnormalities of dyslexics are accompanied by phonological ones. Both phonological and visual skills are required for successful reading and they correlate strongly with each other. These facts lead to the speculation that fundamentally both phonological and visual deficits in dyslexics may be the result of a generalised abnormality of the magnocellular system of neurones in the central nervous system which is responsible for rapid signal processing.

DYSLEXICS' UNSTABLE VISUAL CONTROL

'The letters move around on the page so I can't tell what they're meant to look like or what order they're in.'

'The letters hover over the page.'

'The "e" moves over the "c" so that it looks like an "r".'

These are all remarks which were made by children with reading problems that we have seen. Clearly, what these children describe are unstable visual perceptions. Their symptoms are highly reminiscent of 'oscillopsia', which many patients with uncontrolled eye movements experience. In gross oscillopsia the whole world appears to be in continuous motion, but small involuntary eye movements may cause only small targets such as letters, to appear to move. Thus their descriptions suggest that dyslexic children may lack stable binocular control.

Before describing our evidence that many dyslexic children do indeed have unstable eye control we should examine the question how we normally manage to keep our visual world stable. Why is our mind's eye view of the world stationary, even though our eyes move around all the time? Each time we move our eyes images smear across the retina, yet most of the time the world does not appear to move. The main way in which we determine whether our own eyes or objects in the outside world are moving, is by being able to associate correctly retinal signals about movements of the images with which vision supplies us, with eye movement signals provided by the ocularmotor system. The latter may either be corollary discharges which inform the visual system that the eyes are about to move, or they are derived from feedback provided by orbital proprioceptors, such as the spindles with which the eye muscles are liberally endowed; these report when the eyes have moved. Accurate ocularmotor signals enable the perceptual system to discount any retinal image movements that are merely the consequence of our own eye movements. These associations probably take place mainly in the right posterior parietal cortex (PPC) (Stein, 1990; 1992). During development, retinal and ocular-motor signals must come to be associated correctly with each other, so that object and eye movements can be clearly distinguished. Only if this procedure is successful can we accurately locate objects with respect to ourselves. Clearly, if we cannot distinguish whether our eyes or a target of interest have moved, we would not be able to locate the position of the target accurately. Successful association of retinal and ocularmotor signals is particularly difficult when the eyes are converged at the near point, as is required for reading. This is because under these circumstances the angles of the two eyes with respect to the skull are different; and therefore potentially they can give different indications of the location of the target. The angles of the two eyes must be calibrated in terms of their distance apart in order to compute the direction and distance of the target correctly. Again it seems that the PPC, particularly that on the right hand side in humans, plays a vital role in these calculations (Stein, 1990; 1992).

These considerations make it clear that perceptual stability of the visual world, and hence accuracy of visual localisation, depends on a properly functioning ocularmotor control system to provide stable binocular fixation. Unwanted and unsignalled eye movements would create havoc with stable localisation of targets. We therefore wondered whether the visual symptoms of children with reading problems which I described earlier might be the result of their suffering unstable binocular fixation. So Sue Fowler and I began looking for ocularmotor instability in children with reading difficulties. We have been measuring the binocular fixation stability and vergence control of dyslexic and normal children; and we have correlated our findings with measurements of the accuracy of their visual direction sense, their ability to localise targets accurately and the nature of their visual errors when reading. We have also been investigating techniques designed to improve children's ocularmotor control to see whether improving this might help them to learn to read. If such interventions were successful this would demonstrate clearly that unstable binocular control is a potent cause of children's reading difficulties.

Subjects

Most of our subjects are referred by general practitioners, school medical officers, local educational psychologists, etc. to the Learning Disabilities Clinic, Orthoptic Department, Royal Berkshire Hospital, Reading because they have reading problems. We use the British Ability Scale (BAS) single word reading test to compare with the BAS Similarities and Matrices tests to identify children with severe reading difficulties. Those whose reading is more than two standard deviations behind that expected on the basis of their similarities and matrices scores tests we classify as 'dyslexic'.

We have also studied a large number of unselected primary school children between the ages of 7 and 11, both to provide control groups and to investigate the normal development of stable binocular control. As control groups to compare with the dyslexics we have used either normal readers matched for chronological age, sex and IQ or younger normal readers matched for reading age, sex and IQ. We recruited the control group matched for reading age on the advice of Bradley and Bryant (Bradley and Bryant, 1983) to counter the argument that normal children of the same chronological age may have better binocular control merely because they have had more reading experience than dyslexics. The visual superiority that we found in younger children matched for reading age could not be attributed to their having had more reading experience. Since their reading ages were the same as the dyslexics, so was their reading experience. Hence their visual superiority was likely to be primary, and thus probably a cause of their reading superiority, rather than merely a result of it.

Binocular instability

The main test that we have used to detect binocular instability was the one introduced by Patricia Dunlop for determining the 'dominant', 'leading' or 'reference' eye in a binocular situation (Dunlop, 1972). We have adapted this test to assess whether a child has stable binocular control. In our version of the test (Fowler and Stein, 1980) two fusion slides depicting a house with a central front door are presented separately to the two eyes in a synoptophore.

The child fuses the slides and the synoptophore tubes are then slowly diverged at 1°/sec. The slide seen by the left eye has a post to the right of the door and that seen by the right eye has a different post on the left side of the door. Just before fusion breaks most subjects see one of the posts appear to move towards the door; this is an example of an autokinetic illusion, described by Ogle (1962). When the test is repeated ten times in normal children it is always the post on the same side that appears to move towards the door; and that on the other side never does so, even if the posts are switched round to avoid the child guessing. The subjects that always see the post on the same side appear to move are said to have stable or 'fixed reference'. If a subject reports that different posts appear to move on more than two occasions out of the ten s/he is said to have unstable control. Thus we use the test to determine how consistently a child is able to associate retinal and ocularmotor cues during divergence stress. As mentioned earlier such binocular conditions are particularly relevant to reading because small letters are viewed at about 25 cm with the eyes converged. Also the vergence angle has to be altered slightly with each fixation when reading.

We found that a very high proportion of dyslexic children have unstable binocular control in this test (52–69% in our different studies (Fowler and Stein, 1980; Stein, Riddell and Fowler, 1987) whereas a far smaller proportion of normal readers, whether matched for chronological or reading age, exhibit this abnormality. These results suggest not just an association between unstable binocular control (as measured by the Dunlop test) and poor reading, but, we believe, a clear causal connection. Younger reading age-matched normal readers had better binocular control than the dyslexics; and this enabled them to read as well as the dyslexics even though their reading experience was just as limited and their age was younger (Stein, Riddell and Fowler, 1986).

Normal children

It has nevertheless been argued that our findings are unreliable because our dyslexics were drawn from referrals to an eye hospital, whereas our normal controls were recruited from local primary schools. We therefore carried out a large-scale study of unselected primary school children. We assessed the binocular stability of nearly 1,000 of these children, both good and bad readers (aged 6–12 years) and compared this with their reading (Stein, Riddell and Fowler, 1986). We found that the binocular stability of all the children improved as they grew older. Thus only 54% of 6 year olds had achieved stability, but 70% of 7 year olds and 85% of 9 year olds had done so. So normal children develop binocular stability as they grow older. This developmental effect must always be allowed for in ocularmotor control studies.

We were also able to confirm our previous finding for the clinic sample that instability in the Dunlop test in these unselected primary school children is clearly associated with reading problems. Comparing children of similar ages, those who had stable binocular control had on average 6.3 months higher reading age than those with unstable control. This difference remained significant even after the effects of age and IQ had been allowed for. Thus our finding that a high proportion of clinic-referred dyslexics have unstable binocular control can be generalised to an unselected population of primary school children. Those who had worse binocular control were likely to be worse readers.

We have recently confirmed this result in another way by following a cohort of children from their entry into primary school over the next three years. Those who started with stable binocular control were significantly better readers at the end of the first, second and third years than those who did not; and the rate at which children developed stable control was a strong predictor of their reading progress. The numbers involved in these studies so far are small, but we are adding to them cumulatively.

Eye movement recording

It must be admitted however that our hypothesis is highly controversial. Although our major result has been confirmed by a number of groups (Bishop, Jancey and Steel, 1979; Masters, 1988; Bigelow and McKenzie, 1985; Dunlop, 1979) it has also been heavily criticised (Newman *et al.*, 1985; Bishop, 1989; Evans and Drasdo, 1990). The main reason for this is that the Dunlop test has turned out not to be an easy test to use, especially in inexperienced hands. It requires a child to report accurately his/her perceptions in a complex situation; and the experimenter has to be alert to the common tendency of children to attempt to second guess what they think the tester wants to hear. The random results of their guessing can give rise to a high proportion of false positives (Newman *et al.*, 1985).

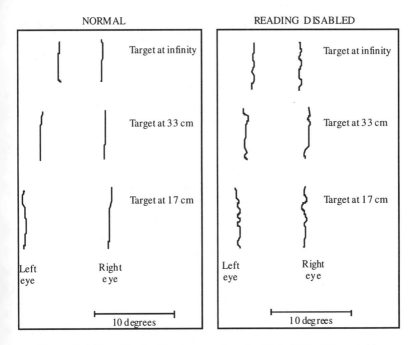

Figure 5.1 Unstable fixation in a reading disabled child with unstable binocular control

We have therefore made many attempts to develop a test which is more objective than the Dunlop test for binocular instability. Using infrared eye movement recordings we have measured children's fixation stability when attempting to fixate small targets at the reading distance (Eden *et al.*, 1993); and we have tried to quantify children's vergence control under different conditions (Stein, Riddell and Fowler, 1988).

Figure 5.1 shows recordings of the positions of the two eyes when two children were attempting to keep their eyes fixed on a small (0.5°) target and viewing distances of 3 metres, 30 and 15 cm (time is upwards). It is easy to see that the reading disabled child with unstable binocular control in the Dunlop test showed considerably larger unwanted eye deviations, especially at the closer distances; these were particularly evident in the left eye. We were able to confirm that dyslexics as a group have more unstable fixation than normal controls; and that this correlates with their Dunlop test responses.

The amplitude of these unwanted eye deviations during attempted fixations were never larger than 1° however. So measuring them routinely in dyslexic children is clearly not a viable proposition. During the Dunlop test the vergence system is put under stress. We have therefore measured the vergence movements made during the Dunlop test to see whether there is a difference between those of children who pass compared with those who fail it (Stein, Riddell and Fowler, 1988). We have been able to show that those who fail the test have a more limited vergence range particularly when diverging from parallel. However because children may be differently motivated to perform this time-consuming and not very exciting test, again it has not proved suitable for routine testing. So far, therefore, we have not been able to develop an eye movement recording procedure which is a clear improvement on the Dunlop test, despite its well-recognised shortcomings.

Visual direction sense

An important prediction of our hypothesis that many dyslexic children suffer visual confusion because of binocular instability is that such confusion should occur not only when they are reading, but also whenever they are required to localise any small target accurately. We have therefore compared the accuracy of the visual direction sense of children who failed the Dunlop test with those who passed it, by means of a computerised dot localisation task (Riddell, Fowler and Stein, 1990). A small target subtending 0.25° was displayed on a VDU screen for 2 sec (long enough for any fixation instability to manifest itself). After a delay of 0.5 sec. a second test spot was then displayed for 200 ms slightly to the left or right of the first. The child's task was to indicate, by pointing, which direction the spot had appeared to move. The distance between target and test spots was adjusted so that the child made approximately 75% correct responses. This was chosen to be halfway between random (50%) and perfect (100%) scores in this two alternative choice dot localisation task. The results were clear and consistent: children with unstable binocular control in the Dunlop test made many more errors for a given separation than either age- or reading age-matched controls.

Moreover, whereas normal children made slightly more errors when the test spot moved to the right of the target in the dot localisation task, the children with unstable binocular control made many more errors on the left. It will be remembered that the fixation stability of these children's left eyes was slightly worse than that on their right. These left/right differences raised the possibility that dyslexic children's visuomotor control on the left might be particularly affected. Such a pattern is reminiscent of patients with lesions of the right posterior parietal cortex.

Visual dyslexic reading errors

Our hypothesis is that binocular control abnormalities cause visual confusion in dyslexic children, and that these give rise to visual reading problems. In order to provide further evidence in favour of this hypothesis we have analysed the kinds of reading errors made by children with unstable compared with stable binocular control, to see whether they provided evidence of their visual origin. Piers Cornelissen classified the errors made by children in the BAS single word reading test. He found the children who failed the Dunlop test tended more often than normals to produce nonsense (nonwords) rather than real words when they attempted words they could not read properly (Cornelissen *et al.*, 1991). We thought that these were probably the result of the children attempting to sound out the confused visual images with which their visual system was presenting them. Likewise Cornelissen found that when visual dyslexics who fail the Dunlop test attempt to spell words which they find difficult, they tend to spell them phonetically. So they make many more phonological regularisation errors than those who pass the Dunlop test.

There is a well-known phonological mechanism which may cause children to make nonword reading errors however. Children with higher phonological ability tend to make nonword errors simply because they try to apply phonological rules to unfamiliar irregular words. So we needed to control for any differences in the children's phonological ability. We therefore designed a study to discover whether children with unstable binocular control made more nonword errors than children of the same reading age with stable binocular control, even if we kept the phonological load on the two groups identical, and also made allowances for differences in the phonological ability of the children. We confirmed that unstable children did indeed make more nonword errors than stable children even under these conditions. Moreover, if print size was increased to reduce the chances of visual confusion, these unstable children decreased the number of nonword errors they made considerably (Cornelissen *et al.*, 1991). These results strongly imply that visual confusion is a significant cause of these children's reading errors.

Cause or effect?

Despite all this evidence, however, it is still argued vehemently by some that there is no causal relationship between unstable binocular control and reading problems. Two alternative possibilities have been put forward: the first is that poor reading is the cause of poor binocular stability rather than the other way round (Bishop, 1989); and the second is that some other neurological abnormality (a *tertiam quid*) causes both. The first possibility is refuted by our evidence that younger normal children reading at the same level as older dyslexics nevertheless have better ocularmotor control than the latter. If their ocularmotor stability were dependent upon their reading, it should be no better than that of the dyslexics.

The second possibility, that some third factor might influence both ocularmotor stability and reading and that therefore binocular stability and reading skill are independent, is unlikely also. First, the strong association that we have shown between binocular instability and the production of nonword errors strongly suggests that the ocularmotor problem causes the reading problem. This conclusion was confirmed by our finding that increasing print size reduced their number of nonword errors (Cornelissen *et al.*, 1991).

Another intervention that we found to reduce significantly the proportion of nonword errors made by children with unstable fixation, was to have them read using only one eye (Cornelissen *et al.*, 1992). These changes, which only affected the visual system, improved their reading; they imply strongly that their visual defect caused this component of their reading problems.

Our rationale for giving these dyslexic children monocular occlusion as a treatment was that if a child is confused by the different views provided by two eyes, then occluding one eye might alleviate the problem. Reading with only one eye turned out not only to reduce the nonword errors made by these children; but if they wore monocularly occluding spectacles for all reading and close work for 6 months the binocular control of over half the unstable children stabilised permanently (Stein and Fowler, 1985). From our large-scale study of normal primary school children we expected 24% of unstable children of this age to become stable spontaneously over 6 months (Stein, Riddell and Fowler, 1986); and we confirmed that this was the proportion of the control group of children whom we gave placebo treatment that achieved stable binocular control. However, with the help of occlusion of the left eye when reading, 51% of unstable dyslexics became stable – a highly significant advantage to those who were occluded.

Achieving binocular stability also had a dramatic effect on these children's reading. In an early pilot study we compared 15 unstable dyslexics treated by means of monocular occlusion with 15 who were not so treated. The 15 who received the occlusion increased their reading age by 12.3 months in the 6 months of observation, whereas the reading of those who were not so treated and who did not gain stable fixation regressed in relation to their age (Fowler and Stein, 1980). In our later placebo controlled trial we gave 60 unstable dyslexics binocularly occluding spectacles and compared their reading progress with that of 40 unstable dyslexics who were given placebo plain spectacles (Stein and Fowler, 1985). Overall the treated dyslexics increased their reading age by an average of 8.4 months in the first 6 months whereas the reading of those who received the placebo spectacles improved by only 6.3 months in the 6 months. As mentioned earlier, about half the unstable dyslexics who received occluding spectacles did not improve their binocular

control. When we compared the 31 unstable dyslexics who did gain
stable ocularmotor control with the help of monocular occlusion
with those who did not, those who gained stable ocularmotor control
increased their reading age by 11.6 months in the first 6 months and
20.6 months in the full year. In contrast those treated with placebo
plain spectacles who did not gain stable binocular control did much
worse, gaining only 5.6 months in their reading age in the first 6
months and 10.6 months in the whole year, i.e., their reading
regressed in relation to their age. What these results strongly suggest
is that correcting children's binocular instability helps them to learn
to read. So we conclude that unstable fixation is indeed a potent
cause of visual confusion, hence of reading problems.

LINK BETWEEN PHONOLOGICAL AND VISUAL
PROBLEMS

One reason why people have found the idea that visual perceptual
deficits have anything to do with reading problems difficult to
accept is that the evidence that most dyslexics have major difficulties
with phonological segmentation is so strong (Bradley and Bryant,
1983; Liberman *et al.*, 1977).

Tests of this ability not only predict reading difficulties
extremely well, but they also correlate highly with reading skill in
normal children. However these facts do not rule out the possibility
that many dyslexic children may suffer visual problems as well. In
most of our studies we have used Bradley and Bryant's rhyming test
(Bradley and Bryant, 1983) to assess the phonological skills of our
subjects; and we have also been fortunate enough to gain access to
Dr. Frank Wood's large Orton dyslexia study data base (Eden *et al.*,
1993) at the Bowman Gray Medical School, Winston Salem, North
Carolina, USA. Thus in two quite distinct groups of children we have
been able to confirm that there is a strong correlation between
phonological and reading abilities. For example, in our Bowman
Gray group of dyslexics and matched controls a test of auditory
analysis skills accounted by itself for over 37% of the variance in the
reading ability of a mixed group of normal and dyslexic children
(Eden, Stein and Wood, 1993).

In addition, however, in many of our studies we have been able to show that there is a strong correlation between children's visual and phonological skills. In the Bowman Gray group the correlation between visual and phonological tests reached 0.4 and this was a highly significant association.

This finding implies not only that phonological and visual skills may share a common neurological mechanism; but they also confirm that very often dyslexics suffer both phonological and visual deficits. We also found however that there was a substantial proportion of the variance in reading ability that could be accounted for only by the particular visual skill in which we are interested, namely binocular stability. This did *not* covary with phonological ability. In the Winston Salem group there was a highly significant 15% of reading variance which was independently predicted by our measures of binocular stability. Thus in most dyslexics visual and phonological disabilities seem to coexist; but beyond this, stable binocular fixation is probably a significant independent contributor to reading skill.

Transient systems?

What neurological mechanisms might underlie the abnormalities of both phonological and visual skills which dyslexics seem to demonstrate? Three lines of enquiry have converged to suggest that a particular class of neurones, the magnocellular system of the central nervous system, may play a crucial role.

Throughout the 1980s Lovegrove and his colleagues published studies (Lovegrove, 1991) which suggested that dyslexics may have slightly reduced performance of the transient, magnocellular, component of their visual processing system. This abnormality may well be the basic cause of dyslexics' binocular instability and visual confusion (see also Lovegrove, this volume).

The visual 'transient' system begins at the large magnocellular ganglion cells in the retina (Shapley, 1990). These project to the magnocellular layers of the lateral geniculate nucleus and to the superior colliculus. Thence they project via the dorsomedial magnocellular pathway through the visual and prestriate cortices to culminate in the posterior parietal cortex (Stein, 1990). This system is widely known as the 'where' pathway because neurones along it respond preferentially to large contour, low contrast, moving targets. It has high contrast sensitivity at low spatial and high temporal frequencies; and it is achromatic, not differentiating between colours. It is thought to signal the location and motion of targets, and therefore to be particularly important for the control of eye and limb movements.

In contrast the parvocellular, 'what', pathway has high spatial and low temporal sensitivity combined with colour selectivity. Its main projection route is via the ventrolateral visual cortical pathway which passes into the inferotemporal cortex. It is believed to help identify objects from the details of their contours and colours.

Measurement of contrast sensitivity over a wide range of spatial frequencies has become a standard method of assessing the function of the visual system (Campbell, 1974). Whereas tests of visual acuity only indicate the performance of the high resolution, high spatial frequency component of visual processing, which is dominated by the parvocellular system, the contrast sensitivity function gives an indication of performance across the whole range of spatial scales. In particular in humans, stimulating at high temporal frequencies using low contrast, low spatial frequency gratings may reveal specific changes in the function of the magnocellular, transient system. Using such stimuli Lovegrove and colleagues have been able to show that most dyslexics exhibit a mild defect of their transient system (Lovegrove, 1991). We have been able to confirm Lovegrove's findings, and we have further shown that this deficit is particularly marked in those with unstable binocular control (Cornelissen, 1993). Hence our current hypothesis is that maldevelopment of the magnocellular system in these children is what causes their binocular instability, hence their visual confusion.

Motion detection is the visual function for which it is generally agreed that the magnocellular system is essential. Hence the psychophysical test which is the most revealing of magnocellular impairments is the measurement of motion sensitivity. We have therefore used random dot kinematograms to assess this in dyslexic adults and children. We recorded what proportion of randomly moving dots had to be moved in the same direction coherently for the subjects to perceive motion. Both the dyslexic adults and children required 3–4% more of the dots to be moving together to perceive motion, than age-matched controls. In other words, the dyslexics were significantly worse at detecting motion than controls

(Cornelissen *et al.*, 1994). Again, therefore, this result supports the idea that at least some disabled readers have a magnocellular deficit.

Another way of demonstrating abnormalities of the magnocellular system is to measure evoked potentials in the visual cortex in response to visual stimuli of low spatial frequency and low contrast. Lovegrove and colleagues (Lovegrove, 1991) and Livingstone *et al.* (1991) have confirmed that many dyslexics show reduced and delayed visual evoked potentials under these conditions. Livingstone *et al.* also examined the brains of five known dyslexics *post mortem* and found that neurones in the magnocellular layers of the lateral geniculate nucleus in these brains appeared to be shrunken and less numerous than normal. This evidence adds to that of Galaburda and colleagues (Galaburda *et al.*, 1985) that there are significant neuroanatomical differences between the brains of normals and dyslexics, again focusing on the possibility that the magnocellular system is the one that is particularly vulnerable.

Posterior Parietal Cortex (PPC)

The highest level of the magnocellular, 'where', system is the PPC. In humans the right PPC is more important for visual localisation; whilst the left probably plays a more important part in phonological processing (Stein, 1990). When the right PPC is damaged by disease in adults a characteristic set of symptoms ensues. The most prominent is left neglect, the inability to direct attention to the left hand side of space or the left hand side of objects. This leads to the patient misjudging the direction, distance and spatial relations of objects, particularly on the left hand side. These are all symptoms which, though much more extreme, are reminiscent of some of the visual problems we have observed in dyslexic children.

So we have been looking for more obvious right parietal symptoms in dyslexic children. The characteristic instability of their left eye during attempts to fixate, and their greater error rate in dot localisation on the left hand side, both mentioned already, are suggestive of right parietal abnormality; and we have found many more indications (Eden *et al.*, 1993). Dyslexics made more errors on the left than normals when copying the Rey figure. They made more errors on the left, when judging the angle of lines with respect to upright. Moreover they made more errors on the left in cancellation tasks. In these the subject has to strike out with a pencil all targets of a certain type amongst a jumble of similar ones. Finally many dyslexics drew clocks like the one shown in Figure 5.2, tending to cram all the figures into the right hand side and leave the left side empty. In patients with right-sided parietal lesions this is a classic sign of 'neglect'. The tendency of dyslexics to make more errors on the left in all these tests suggests that there may indeed be something abnormal about the right PPC of many dyslexic children.

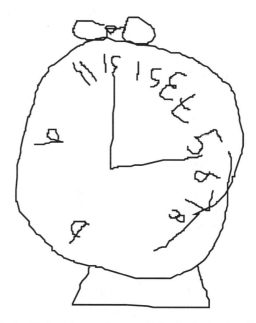

Figure 5.2 Left-sided neglect and reversed figures in the drawing of a clock by a dyslexic child with unstable binocular control

Impaired temporal processing

It should not be forgotten that there is equally strong evidence that most dyslexics have left-sided, linguistic problems as well. Paula Tallal and her colleagues have published a series of studies in developmental dysphasics over the last 20 years which show, that like the visual problems of developmental dyslexics described in this chapter, the phonological difficulties of dysphasics are not confined to the linguistic domain; instead they are part of a more generalised defect of auditory analysis. She has shown that dysphasics take longer than normals to be able to distinguish between two tones presented in rapid sequence (Tallal and Mishkin, 1982). Likewise their voice onset time (VOT) is prolonged compared with normals.

Interestingly from our point of view, she has also found that dysphasics' ability to discriminate small symbols (not letters) presented visually in a rapid sequence is impaired. Many such dysphasics go on to become dyslexics. Angela Fawcett, Rod Nicolson and colleagues (see chapter by Fawcett and Nicolson, this volume) have found that dyslexics show signs of impaired rapid signal processing in several other sensory and motor domains. They have a longer latency P300 auditory evoked potential in an auditory 'oddball' paradigm; dyslexics have slower choice reaction time, despite normal simple reaction times; they have higher two-point touch thresholds but normal sensitivity to a single point; and they have a tendency to fall over when balancing on a beam if blindfolded or given a secondary cognitive task to perform. All these findings can be interpreted in terms of impairment of rapid signal processing in the auditory, somaesthetic and motor systems; not in their peripheral pathways, but in the centres responsible for stimulus and response categorisation.

The parallels between the signal processing deficits of dyslexics in different sensory and motor domains are clearly striking; they prompt us to speculate that they may all share a common origin. The very different techniques of genetic analysis suggest the same thing. Dyslexia is strongly heritable, as are reading and its component skills, visual and phonological analysis (Olson *et al.*, 1989). The heritability of somaesthetic and motor skills has not been studied in the same way. Nevertheless a plausible hypothesis is that what is inherited in normals as well as dyslexics are not specific visual, auditory or other skills but the general ability to perform rapid neuronal processing operations. These are required for all the rapid visual, auditory and articulatory sequencing tasks that are important for reading.

My final speculation is therefore that a genetically based defect of rapid signal processing is the fundamental cause of dyslexic problems. So far such a defect has only been clearly shown for the visual magnocellular system. But magnocellular neurones contribute not only to visual processing but also to every other function of the nervous system; auditory, somaesthetic and motor. The development of magnocellular neurones probably involves the expression of a common surface active molecule. Clearly if immunological action *in utero* attacked this surface active molecule specific to large neurones this would damage magnocellular systems throughout the brain, and give rise to just such a combination of visual phonological and motor disorders as we see in dyslexics. The multidimensional nature of dyslexics' problems could thus be explained by a single underlying molecular mechanism occurring during development.

REFERENCES

Bigelow, E.R. and McKenzie, B.E. (1985). Unstable ocular dominance and reading ability. *Perception, 14*, 329–335.

Bishop, D.V.M. (1989). Unstable vergence control and dyslexia – a critique. *British Journal of Ophthalmology, 73*, 223–245.

Bishop, D.V.M., Jancey, C. and Steel, A.McP. (1979). Orthoptic status and reading disability. *Cortex, 15*, 659–666.

Bradley, L. and Bryant, P. (1983). Categorising sounds and learning to read – a causal connection. *Nature, 301*, 419–421.

Campbell, F.W. (1974). The transmission of spatial information through the visual system. In F.O. Schmidt (Ed.), *The Neurosciences 3rd Study Program* (pp. 95–123). Cambridge, MA: MIT Press.

Cornelissen, P. (1993). Fixation, contrast sensitivity and children's reading. In S.E. Wright (Ed.), *Studies in Visual Information Processing* (pp. 139–163). Amsterdam: North-Holland.

Cornelissen, P., Bradley, L., Fowler, M.S. and Stein, J.F. (1991). What children see affects how they read. *Developmental Medicine and Child Neurology, 33*, 755–762.

Cornelissen, P., Bradley, L., Fowler, M.S. and Stein, J.F. (1992). Covering one eye affects how some children read. *Developmental Medicine and Child Neurology, 34*, 296–304.

Cornelissen, P., Richardson, A., Mason, A., and Stein, J.F. (1994). Coherent motion detection in reading–disabled children and adults. *Vision Research* (in press).

Dunlop, P. (1972). Dyslexia: The orthoptic approach. *Australian Journal of Orthoptics, 12*, 16–20.

Dunlop, P. (1979). Orthoptic management of learning disability. *British Orthoptic Journal, 36,* 25–35.

Eden, G.F., Stein, J.F. and Wood, F.B. (1993). Visuospatial ability and language processing in reading disabled and normal children. In S.E. Wright (Ed.), *Studies in Visual Information Processing* (pp. 321–337). Amsterdam: North-Holland.

Evans, B.J.W. and Drasdo, N. (1990). Ophthalmic factors in dyslexia. *Ophthalmic and Physiological Optics, 10,* 123–132.

Fowler, S. and Stein, J. (1980). Visual dyslexia. *British Orthoptic Journal, 37,* 11.

Galaburda, A.M., Sherman, G.F., Rosen, G.D., Abotiz, F. and Geschwind, N. (1985). Developmental dyslexia: Four consecutive patients with cortical anomalies. *Annals of Neurology, 18,* 222–233.

Liberman, I.Y., Shankweiler, D., Liberman, A.M., Fowler, C. and Fischer, F.W. (1977). Phonetic segmentation and recoding in the beginning reader. In A.S. Reber and D. Scarborough (Eds.), *Reading: Theory and practice.* Hillsdale, NJ: Lawrence Erlbaum Associates.

Livingstone, M.S., Rosen, G.D., Drislane, F.W. and A.M. Galaburda (1991). Physiological and anatomical evidence for a magnocellular defect in developmental dyslexia. *Proceedings of the National Academy of Sciences of the United States of America, 88,* 7943–7947.

Lovegrove, W. (1991). Spatial frequency processing in normal and dyslexic readers. In J. Stein (Ed.), *Visual Dyslexia,* vol.13. *Vision and Visual Dysfunction.* London: Macmillan Press.

Masters, M.C. (1988). Orthoptic management of visual dyslexia. *British Orthoptic Journal, 45,* 40–48.

Newman, S.P., Karle, H., Wadsworth, J.F., Archer, R., Hockly, R. and Rogers, P. (1985). Ocular dominance, reading and spelling: A reassessment of a measure associated with specific reading difficulties. *Journal of Research in Reading, 8,* 127–138.

Ogle, K.N. (1962). The optic space sense. In H. Davson, (Ed.), *The Eye* vol. ix. New York: Academic Press.

Olson, R.K., Wise, B., Conners, F., Rack, J. and Fulker, D. (1989). Specific deficits in component reading and language skills: Genetic and environmental influences. *Journal of Learning Disabilities, 22,* 339–348.

Riddell, P., Fowler, M.S. and Stein, J.F. (1990). Spatial discrimination in children with poor vergence control. *Perceptual and Motor Skills, 70,* 707–718.

Shapley, R. (1990). Parallel visual processing pathways. *Annual Review of Psychology, 41,* 635–638.

Stein, J.F. (1990). Representation of egocentric space in the Posterior Parietal Cortex. *Quarterly Journal of Experimental Psychology, 74,* 583–606.

Stein, J.F. (1992). Representation of egocentric space in the posterior parietal cortex. *Behavioural and Brain Sciences, 15*, 691–703.

Stein, J.F. and Fowler, M.S. (1985). Effect of monocular occlusion on visuomotor perception and reading in dyslexic children. *The Lancet*, 13 July, 69–73.

Stein, J.F., Riddell, P. and Fowler, M.S. (1986). The Dunlop test and reading in primary school children. *British Journal of Ophthalmology, 70*, 317.

Stein, J.F., Riddell, P. and Fowler, M.S. (1987). Fine binocular control in dyslexic children. *Eye, 1*, 433–438.

Stein, J.F., Riddell, P. and Fowler, M.S. (1988). Disordered vergence eye movement control in dyslexic children. *British Journal of Ophthalmology, 72*, 162–166.

Tallal, P. and Mishkin, M. (1982). Defects of non–verbal auditory perception in children with developmental aphasia. *Nature, 241*, 468–469.

Vellutino, F.R. (1987). Dyslexia. *Scientific American, 256*, 20–27.

CHAPTER 6

Speed of processing, motor skill, automaticity and dyslexia

Angela J. Fawcett and Roderick I. Nicolson

INTRODUCTION

In the five preceding chapters of this volume we have seen clear evidence that dyslexic children show deficits in phonological skill and in visual skill, together with tantalising suggestions that these may derive, at least in part, from problems in rapid processing of auditory and/or visual information. For this sixth chapter we commissioned ourselves to attempt to summarise the literature on speed of processing deficits and on motor skills in dyslexia. We have also taken the opportunity to review theoretical work on the acquisition of skill, in that we believe that a skill acquisition framework provides a valuable alternative perspective for considering the range of difficulties suffered by dyslexic people.

The chapter is organised as follows: first, we review the literature on speed of processing and dyslexia, completing the section with one of our studies which shows clear evidence of reduced speed of processing even in a task which has no overt or covert phonological component. Like many other dyslexia researchers, and the contributors to this volume, we conclude that there is clear evidence both of phonological deficits and of speed of processing deficits in dyslexia. Next we review the literature on motor skill, again concluding that there is consistent evidence of difficulty, especially for younger children. We note, however, that the skills under consideration have a strong learned or maturational aspect, and suggest that the difficulties might arise from abnormalities in the general learning process, rather than the specific skills investigated. Following an overview of current theories of skill acquisition, we note that automatisation is one of the key concepts in acquisition of fluency in a skill. We then propose the twin hypotheses that dyslexic children suffer from a general deficit in the ability to automatise skills (the Dyslexic Automatisation Deficit hypothesis), but that normally they are able in many circumstances to mask the automatisation deficit by means of working harder (our Conscious Compensation hypothesis). The theory was tested by investigating the ability to balance without wobbling, and was strongly supported by our findings that dyslexic children showed clear balance deficits when prevented from concentrating on their balance (by a distracting task or being blindfolded), but that in normal circumstances their balance appeared normal. We finish the chapter by briefly reviewing two experiments on long-term learning of skill, in which we established that dyslexic children are able to automatise a skill, but their initial performance is impaired, their apparent rate of learning (and especially elimination of errors) may be reduced and their final 'quality' of performance is impaired. We consider briefly the implications of these results for the concept of automatisation deficit, but defer further theoretical discussion to our final chapter, which reports on more recent work.

SPEED OF PROCESSING AND DYSLEXIA

Although developmental dyslexia is generally characterised by unexpected problems in learning to read, one of the more striking features of the performance profile for dyslexic children is an impairment in speed in almost any skill. Many dyslexic children are able to overcome their early reading problems in terms of word reading accuracy, but performance for even these remediated dyslexics remains slow and laboured (see Yap and van der Leij, this volume). Anecdotal reports suggest this lack of fluency may characterise dyslexic performance across a range of skills. For instance, Miles (1983) draws on several case histories, citing the anomalous performance of dyslexic children who fail on mundane mental arithmetic tasks which must be completed within an allotted time-span, yet are capable of identifying complex relationships on a reasoning task. Miles argues that any requirement to perform a task in 'paced' conditions (i.e., at the experimenter's pace not the child's pace) has a detrimental effect on the performance of dyslexic people, regardless of age. A range of experimental evidence clearly shows more marked deficits in literacy subskills for dyslexic children under paced or timed tests than under more relaxed conditions (e.g., Ellis and Miles, 1981; Seymour, 1986). The pervasive ramifications of such a deficit impinge on the everyday life of the dyslexic, constantly struggling to keep pace with the demands.

This impairment may be clearly seen in analysis of scores on the Wechsler Intelligence Scale for Children (WISC-R: Wechsler, 1976), an intelligence test widely used in the diagnosis of dyslexia. Dyslexic children's performance on the individual components typically shows an abnormally spiky profile, reflecting a distinctive pattern of strengths and weaknesses. Following early work by Newton and Thomson (1976) several researchers have noted the characteristic form that this profile takes, with deficit in one or more of the following subtests: Arithmetic (a test of mental arithmetic including tables), Coding (the transcription of a sequence of arbitrary symbols), Information (a test of general knowledge) and Digit span (a memory span test) – the aptly named ACID profile.

The ACID profile illustrates the interplay between phonological difficulties and reduced speed of processing. Problems in Information may initially be attributed to low vocabulary which in turn derives from phonological problems, subsequently exacerbated by difficulties in picking up information from the written word. Digit span problems have been attributed to a deficient phonological input store (Gathercole and Baddeley, 1990), and this in turn may arise from deficient lexical representations (Hulme, Maughan and Brown, 1991). Miles (1983) has suggested that arithmetic problems derive from difficulties in learning associations and that this may reflect the underlying problem of 'verbal labelling', particularly under timed conditions. On the other hand, problems in Coding are less naturally explained under a pure phonological deficit and seem to implicate speed of processing. Thomson (1991) suggests that coding is a 'practical' skill, dependent on a combination of speed, visual and motor co-ordination in the presence of sustained effort. Regardless of the precise task demands of Coding, it is clear that processing speed is an important component, and therefore it appears that speed may well be an important contributory factor on several of the specific weaknesses of dyslexic children. We turn now to the literature directly assessing processing speed in dyslexia.

Naming speed deficits in dyslexia

There is an extensive literature on deficits in speed of access to the spoken word, initially discovered using the 'rapid automatised naming' (RAN) test (Denckla and Rudel, 1976). This test involves the rapid sequential naming of 50 familiar stimuli presented together on a card. The authors showed that dyslexic children were slower even than reading age-matched controls to name colours, pictures, digits and letters. It has been suggested that a naming deficit may be specific to dyslexia, rather than common to the garden-variety poor reader (Wolf and Obregon, 1992), or to attention-deficit disorder (Felton *et al.*, 1987). This naming deficit has been consistently replicated (e.g., Swanson, 1987), and is evident not only with visual stimuli but also with auditory presentations and the naming of objects identified by touch (Rudel, Denckla and Broman, 1981). More recently, in a longitudinal study of pre-readers, Wolf (1991) has identified speed of naming as one of the most critical predictors of later reading performance, even after controlling for vocabulary level. She also demonstrated a direct relationship between speed deficits in naming letters and numbers and severity of impairment in the dyslexic case studies presented. Continued problems with the RAN have been identified with both digits and letters in adolescent and adult dyslexics (see e.g., Denckla and Rudel, 1976; Bowers, Steffy and Tate, 1988).

Results are often less clear-cut with discrete trial (rather than continuous) presentations, reflecting again the distinction between unpaced and paced procedures (Wolf, 1991). However, Wolff and his colleagues (Wolff, Michel and Ovrut, 1990a) have recently demonstrated an increase in error rate in response to flashed presentations of objects and colours for dyslexic adolescents and adults. This deficit in accuracy was evident in comparison with both matched controls and learning disabled children without reading difficulties, and correlated highly with naming latencies on a (continuous) RAN presentation.

Study 1: Speed of simple reaction and choice reaction

It is therefore established that any task which demands continuous speeded access to lexical information will demonstrate deficiencies in speed of information processing in dyslexic subjects. In view of the central role of information processing speed in cognitive skills, it is particularly surprising that until recently there appeared to be no reports of direct investigations of speed in the literature on dyslexia. Consequently, we designed a series of experiments explicitly to test 'raw' processing speed, uncontaminated by the effects of linguistic competence (see Nicolson and Fawcett, 1994, for full details). Our research strategy was to investigate speed of information processing using a series of simpler and simpler reaction time tasks in the hope that at some point we would find a cut-off where tasks of lesser complexity would show no deficit, whereas more complex tasks would result in a deficit – that is, the point at which performance first became abnormal. If this point lay where lexical material first appeared, this would provide further strong converging evidence for the phonological deficit hypothesis, whereas a continuing deficit with non-lexical material would indicate that the underlying cause lay deeper.

We established in pilot studies that dyslexic children showed the expected speed deficit in linguistically-based tasks. Consequently, in an attempt to find normal performance, we administered increasingly simple tasks – lexical decision, choice reaction, and finally simple reaction to a tone. First, in the lexical decision task, subjects were presented auditorily with a word (or, equally probably, a morphologically valid nonword created by altering the first consonant) and had to say as quickly as possible Yes (if it was a word, such as *shop*) or No (if it was a nonword, such as *thop*). We were interested in the speed of their response. In both reaction time experiments, the children sat with a single button in their preferred hand, and their task was to press it as quickly as possible whenever they heard a low tone. In the simple reaction (SRT) task, no other tone was ever presented, but in the selective choice reaction (SCRT) task, there was an equal probability of a high tone being presented. If the high tone was presented, the subject simply had to do nothing. These are established experimental tasks, introduced by Donders well over a century ago. His rationale was that the only difference between the tasks was the need to classify the stimulus before responding in the SCRT trials, and he argued that subtracting the simple reaction time (SRT) from the SCRT time gave an estimate of 'stimulus classification' time. Most subsequent research has preferred the choice reaction (for a two-choice reaction the subject has two buttons, and presses the left button for the low tone and the right button for the high tone, say). Unfortunately, dyslexic children have problems with distinguishing left and right (Miles, 1983), and so any deficit in a choice reaction might plausibly be attributed to left/right confusions. The comparison between SCRT and SRT is not subject to this type of problem since only one hand is used.

Like other researchers in the area, we have found that one of the major problems of working with dyslexic children is the heterogeneity of their performance. These differences are compounded by qualitative differences in the overlay of learned skills, and the maturation process itself. In order to control for these factors, we monitored longitudinal changes by using two age groups of dyslexic children (mean ages 15 and 11 years), together with both reading age match and chronological age match control groups (mean ages 15, 11 and 8 years). We shall refer to the dyslexic and control groups as Dys 15 and Dys 11; and Cont 15, Cont 11 and Cont 8, respectively. Note that the Cont 11 group served as the chronological age match for the Dys 11 group and also as the reading age match for the Dys 15 group. The Cont 8 group served as reading age controls for Dys 11. The results for simple reaction, selective choice reaction and lexical access are shown in Figure 6.1, plotted on the same graph to allow easy comparison.

On the simple reactions the older children, whether dyslexic or control, were significantly faster than the 11-year-old children, who were faster than the 8-year-old children. There was a significant effect of age but not of dyslexia. When we compared the two dyslexic groups with their reading age controls we found an effect of both age and dyslexia. In this case, however, the dyslexic groups were *faster* than their reading age controls. This pattern of results shows the well-known improvement in reaction time with age, but demonstrates no effect of dyslexia whatsoever.

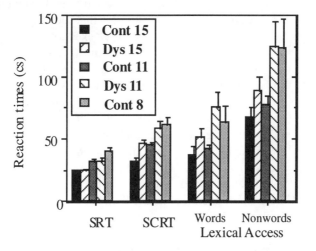

Figure 6.1 Reaction times for simple reactions, selective choice reactions and lexical access

On the selective choice reactions, by contrast, there were highly significant differences between the groups. The dyslexic children performed significantly more slowly and less accurately than their age-matched controls, and at the level of their reading age-matched controls.

For lexical decisions the dyslexic children again performed significantly slower than their age-matched controls, and at the level of their reading age-matched controls, with no difference in accuracy. However, a further series of analyses on the lexical decision data was needed to check that the effect we had found did not derive from a subset of the items presented. Accordingly, we collapsed the data across the subjects in the groups, to perform a 'by item' analysis. This showed a similar pattern of results to our standard analysis, but interestingly enough, a stronger pattern of results emerged, with the dyslexic groups now significantly worse than their reading age controls on the words.

The results of this study are particularly interesting; normal performance for the dyslexic children on the simple reaction time suggests that not only their cognitive and metacognitive skills but also their motor responses are unimpaired. Consequently the most likely locus of the dyslexics' deficit appears to be the time needed to classify the stimulus ('perceptual impairment'). On the other hand, one might equally plausibly suggest that although the stimuli are classified just as quickly, the 'central executive' simply takes longer to make the correct decision ('central executive impairment'). In practice, of course there is very little to choose between the two explanations, though auditory evoked potentials to the tones may be able to provide some useful information on the source of the deficit. In fact a recent study of the SCRT task in a small group of our older dyslexics and controls showed that it was possible to differentiate the groups blind on the basis of their P300 response (Fawcett *et al.*, 1993). The P300 is held to be an index of stimulus classification speed, uncontaminated by response selection factors (Coles, Gratton and Fabiani, 1990).

Our initial motivation was to present a series of experiments testing 'raw' processing speed, unaffected by the effects of linguistic competence. It is important therefore to link these results back to the literature on impairments in speed of linguistic processing in dyslexic children. Interestingly enough, in a series of studies of language disabled children, Paula Tallal (e.g., 1980) has shown deficits in rapid temporal processing of linguistic information in terms of both perception and production. Tallal has shown that children with language delay have problems in processing rapidly changing information, once it passes a critical threshold for speed of presentation. The data she presented were based on a conditioning (training) paradigm, in which children were trained to respond to two different steady-state tones of different frequencies, presented in rapid succession. The basis of the deficit for the language disabled group seemed to be in simply discriminating the tones at rapid rates of presentation, leading to failure to sequence them successfully. Using this repetition test, Tallal and colleagues were able to differentiate successfully 98% of her language delayed sample from controls (Tallal, Stark and Mellit, 1985).

Consider the implications of a deficit in rapid processing of the simplest auditorily presented information in terms of the competence of the developing child. At each stage in development, a series of small deficits in speed of processing may cumulate into a substantial impairment. This is typical of the pattern of results obtained, for instance, in the naming studies, in performance on the Coding subtest of the WISC, in low scores on repetition of digits, in fact on any task in which the child must maintain a paced performance. We have identified an underlying non-phonological deficit in stimulus classification speed, consistent with speed impairments in either the classification or central decision processes. There are intriguing parallels here with the problems in processing rapidly presented visual information through the transient system which Lovegrove (this volume) describes.

The children Tallal identified have a good deal in common with the dyslexic children studied here, many of whom show some degree of subtle impairment in language. Nevertheless, it is important also to consider that the discrimination skills we are talking about must be learned in just the same way as any other. Improvements in the performance of young children on reaction time tests can be achieved with systematic training (Nicolson, 1982) suggesting that the task taps the listener's level of perceptual learning (Tomblin and Quinn, 1983). Furthermore, a computer manipulation of the rate of change of the temporal characteristics of speech sounds resulted in a significant enhancement of speech perception in the language delayed group (Tallal, 1983). Further research is needed to identify whether we are dealing here with a biologically determined limitation in temporal processing, an impairment in learning, or some combination of the two deficits. As discussed in the following section, we had *a priori* grounds for predicting an impairment in learning.

MOTOR SKILLS AND DYSLEXIA

The studies reported in this section originally derived from longitudinal research on 23 dyslexic children who were studied in depth over several years as part of Fawcett's doctoral research (Fawcett, 1990). In this research a fascinating picture emerged both of the current capabilities of the children and the ways their abilities had changed over the years. In the time since diagnosis, the reading abilities of the dyslexic children had diverged, so that ten were technically 'remediated', in that their reading performance had improved to within the normal range (within one year of their chronological age), whereas the remainder had lost further ground, most lagging three years or more behind normal performance.

Interestingly enough, although the single word reading of the remediated group had become as good as that of control children, any more sensitive analyses suggested a continued lack of fluency – their reading was more laboured, more prone to error, more susceptible to interference from other tasks. This incomplete mastery is a characteristic of dyslexic performance, sometimes established difficulties, such as problems catching a ball (Haslum, 1989) or tying shoelaces (Augur, 1985) but more often anecdotal reports such as tendencies to being distractible, absent-minded or accident-prone. Theoretical accounts of the acquisition of skill (Fitts and Posner, 1967; Anderson, 1982) attribute fluency in performance to 'automatisation' of the skill – the gradual reduction in the need for conscious attentive control of performance, with an accompanying increase in speed and efficiency coupled with a decreased likelihood of breakdown under stress. The studies presented here were designed to examine the performance of the dyslexic group on motor skills for further signs of this incomplete mastery in a realm explicitly divorced from their known areas of deficit in language and reading. We shall first review briefly the existing findings on motor skills, then review theoretical analyses of acquisition of skill, and then outline the findings of the studies.

First of all let us consider fine motor skills. Of course, one of the most evident signs of abnormality in dyslexia is the often quite atrocious quality of handwriting (Miles, 1983). Although most theorists have concentrated rather more on the atrocious quality of the spellings conveyed therein, it must be emphasised that handwriting is a motor skill, and (apart from an understandable reluctance to avoid illegibility) there is no obvious reason to link handwriting skill with phonological skills. There is also evidence that young dyslexic children up to the age of 8 have difficulty in tying shoelaces (Benton, 1978; Miles, 1983). Deficits have also been noted in young dyslexic children in copying (for example, on the Bender Gestalt, which measures grapho-motor control in the copying of nine geometric shapes and later drawing them from memory (e.g.,

Benton, 1978; Rudel, 1985). Understandably, this led to the theory in the 1970s that this reflected some basic visual deficit. The underlying cause of this anomaly was, however, pinpointed in a study by Rudel (1985), who showed that dyslexic children were good at judging which drawing was a more accurate copy, despite their evident difficulties in copying. There have also been some suggestions that deficits in fine motor skills – for instance, grasping a pen for writing – may represent an emotional reaction to anticipated frustration (Denckla, 1985).

There is some reported evidence of gross motor coordination problems in young dyslexic children, for instance Augur (1985) reported early coordination difficulties in skills such as bicycle riding and swimming. In an extensive longitudinal study, the British Births Cohort study, Haslum (1989) examined aspects of health in a cohort of 12,905 children at each age. As part of the testing procedure for the 10-year-old children, selected items of the Bangor Dyslexia test (Miles, 1983) were administered, allowing dyslexic children to be identified, and thereby allowing analysis of those factors which were highly associated with dyslexia at birth, 5 years and 10 years. In brief, the tests that correlated most highly with dyslexia were: balancing on one leg, walking backwards, sorting matches, and a graphaesthetic task (reproducing a shape drawn on the back of the hand out of sight of the subject); together with family history, birth history and childhood diseases. Two motor skills tasks emerged among the 6 variables significant at age 10, namely failure to throw a ball up, clap several times and catch the ball ($p < .001$) and failure to walk backwards in a straight line for six steps ($p < .01$).

There is also a substantial literature on dyslexic performance on tapping and related finger movements. For example, Denckla (1985) and Rudel (1985) have identified deficits in movements such as toe tapping and successive opposition of fingers and thumbs, while Urion and colleagues (1987) also identified difficulties in synkinesis and mirror movements in young dyslexic children. In addition to strong evidence of phonological deficits, in young children with dyslexia there is also considerable evidence for a deficit in motor skills in speed of tapping, heel–toe placement, rapid successive finger opposition and accuracy in copying (Denckla, 1985). Children with dyslexia, Denckla suggested, are characterised by a 'non-specific developmental awkwardness', so that even those children with dyslexia who show reasonable athletic ability are poorly co-ordinated. This awkwardness is typically outgrown by puberty (Rudel, 1985), leading Denckla and Rudel to argue for a maturational lag in the 'motor analyser' which programmes timed sequential movements (Denckla, 1985). Moreover, they suggested that these deficits are primarily in the acquisition of new tasks, which is typically awkward and effortful, but once the skill is successfully acquired, dyslexic performance is essentially normal. Interestingly, however, Wolff and his colleagues (1984; 1990b) were able to identify motor skill deficits persisting into adolescence. The task they used involved the reproduction of the rhythm of a metronome, tapping in time with the beat for 30 seconds, and continuing to tap in the same rhythm for a further 30 seconds once the metronome had stopped. They identified a speed threshold at which performance broke down in terms of accuracy in bimanual or intermanual performance in 12–13-year-old dyslexics with language deficits. Wolff and his colleagues argued that impaired interlimb coordination underlay the poor performance of retarded readers at a speed threshold. At a slow rate, both retarded readers and controls performed adequately. They suggested, however, that *speeded* movements interfere with the efficient sequential organisation of motor patterns.

There is also considerable evidence that children with dyslexia are impaired in articulatory skill (Catts, 1986; 1989; Snowling, 1981; Stanovich, 1988; Wolff *et al.*, 1984; 1990c), but it is not clear whether this is caused primarily by a phonological or a motor skill deficit in the rate or accuracy of articulation. The deficit was originally identified as errors in the repetition of polysyllabic or nonsense words, coupled with error-free performance in the repetition of simple high-frequency words for young children with dyslexia (Snowling, 1981). Similarly, Stanovich (1988) established that poor readers up to age 10 showed deficits in their speed of repetition of simple couplets, leading him to argue for a developmental lag in motor timing control. For adolescents with dyslexia, Wolff and his colleagues identified problems in rapid paced repetition of sequences (Wolff *et al.*, 1984; 1990c). The task used in the latter study was the repetition of the sequence *pa-ta-ka*, entrained to the beat of a metronome. Wolff found that his subjects had difficulty in constructing a fluent speech rhythm, particularly at the faster speeds. Similar deficits were found for this age group in repetition of simple and complex phrases (Catts, 1986; 1989). However, although Brady, Shankweiler and Mann (1983) found that 8-year-old children with dyslexia were significantly slower and less accurate in repeating polysyllables and nonsense words, they found no impairment in accuracy or speed of a single repetition of high-frequency monosyllables. In summary, there is evidence that children with dyslexia are slower and more error-prone on complex articulation tasks, but their performance appears to be normal on simple, familiar words.

It is clear, therefore, that there are consistent indications that dyslexic children have problems with motor skill in addition to their problems in phonological skill. However, a study by Tallal and Stark (1982) showed no impairment in balance or motor control coordination for 7–9-year-old dyslexic children without concomitant language difficulties. Most researchers, therefore, would concur with Rudel's (1985) general conclusion that motor skill deficits tend to be with newly acquired skills and (except, perhaps, for complex, time-dependent skills) to be largely outgrown by the age of 9–10 years.

It should be noted, however, that, although difficulties in motor skill are clearly not as disabling as the language-related difficulties, they also need explaining, and may be just as valuable in identifying the underlying cause. Furthermore, given that motor skill deficits are most marked in early childhood, such deficits might prove valuable at an age before reading-based measures are available for diagnostic purposes. It is therefore surprising that little work has been undertaken recently to investigate the reasons for the association between motor skill deficit and dyslexia. The possible reasons for the association are perhaps best approached via a theoretical analysis of the processes of motor skill development.

THEORIES OF MOTOR SKILL DEVELOPMENT

A very influential account of motor skill development was derived by Paul Fitts (Fitts and Posner, 1967). In brief, he analysed the learning process into three stages: the cognitive stage, in which the basic task requirements are determined; the associative phase, in which a method for carrying out the requirements is worked out; and the autonomous phase, in which the task is carried out more and more smoothly, with less and less need for conscious attention. To take the example of learning to drive a car, if one's objective is to select third gear, the cognitive phase includes knowing when to select third gear, what the gear stick layout is, what the function of the clutch pedal is, and so on. The associative phase involves the learning of the sequence – release accelerator pedal, depress clutch pedal, move gearstick up across and up again, release clutch pedal, depress accelerator pedal. However, this process initially needs a great deal of conscious monitoring, to the extent that the beginner actually has to watch his/her hand moving the gearstick, to the potential peril of those in the vicinity! With extended practice, rather than six sequential actions, the whole procedure becomes a single smooth composite action, requiring little or no conscious monitoring. The skill has become autonomous, or automatic.

About a decade later, in a programmatic investigation of the processes of skill acquisition, Shiffrin and Schneider (1977) established that with prolonged training an arbitrary cognitive skill could become automatic, but only if the learning conditions were appropriate. In particular, they distinguished between 'consistent mapping', in which the required action to a given stimulus remained the same throughout training, and 'varied mapping' in which the required action to a given stimulus was varied randomly throughout the training. They demonstrated that consistent mapping was a prerequisite for the development of automaticity, and distinguished between two types of process:

(1) *Controlled Processing*: Requires attentional control, uses up working memory capacity and is often serial. It is relatively easy to set up, modify and use in novel situations. It is used to facilitate long-term learning of all kinds (including automatisation).

(2) *Automatic Processing*: Once learned in long-term memory it operates independently of the subject's control and uses no working memory resources. It does not require attention (though it may attract it if the training is appropriate). It is acquired through consistent mapping. Targets can acquire the ability to attract attention and initiate responses automatically, immediately and independent of other memory loads.

Anderson's ACT* model (1982; 1989) of the acquisition of skill probably represents the most influential current view of cognitive learning, and since it may be traced back directly to Fitts and Posner's (1967) account of motor learning, it forms a reasonable framework for the analysis of both motor and cognitive skill. ACT* suggests that the learning process may be conceptualised as three broad stages (analogous to the stages of Fitts and Posner). Declarative knowledge (e.g., the task requirements) must be acquired initially. This declarative knowledge must then be 'proceduralised' by a 'knowledge compilation' process consequent upon successful performance, turning it into a production rule format which can be used to carry out the requirements. The production rules may subsequently be tuned by extended practice, thus making them more efficient. Automatisation occurs in this final stage, making the procedures less dependent upon working memory, and less susceptible to interference.

One of Anderson's achievements was to demonstrate that this theory of learning could be applied not just to 'motor' tasks such as studied by Fitts and Posner but also to a range of cognitive skills, including geometrical reasoning, computer programming, development of language and letter recognition. In skills such as chess, the declarative stage (learning how the pieces move, what their value is, the rules of the game, common openings etc.) can take years, and is obviously interleaved with the acquisition of procedural skills such as learning to win with rook and king against king. In motor skills such as learning to write a letter 'b', the declarative component presumably comprises the knowledge of the shape of the letter, plus the preferred order of pen strokes. For a skilled writer attempting to write an unfamiliar letter, say a 'ψ', the necessary subskills for writing the individual components are presumably highly learned, and the major difficulty is the declarative learning problem of identifying and remembering what the segments are. It may be seen why studies of learning are so fraught with difficulty. For even a moderately complex task there is a range of possible methods, each involving previously learned skills, each of which may be more or less automatised.

The 'Dyslexic Automatisation Deficit' and 'Conscious Compensation' hypotheses

It is evident that a skill acquisition perspective should be of use in analyses of reading problems. Consider the conclusions of a recent detailed overview and analysis of the teaching of reading: 'Laboratory research indicates that the most critical factor beneath fluent word reading is the ability to recognise letters, spelling patterns, and whole words effortlessly, automatically and visually. The central goal of all reading instruction – comprehension – depends critically on this ability.' (Adams, 1990, p. 54). The reason that theorists have not seriously considered general skill acquisition as a viable framework is that it fails to explain the apparent specificity of the deficits in dyslexia. If they have a general problem in learning, why do dyslexic children not show problems in *all* skills, cognitive and motor?

In our approach to this difficulty we were encouraged first by the observation that, whatever skill theorists had examined carefully (with the single exception of spatial skills), a deficit had been observed in dyslexic children. Furthermore, careful observation of dyslexic children suggests that, although they appear to be behaving normally, they show unusual lapses of concentration and get tired more quickly than normal when performing a skill (Augur, 1985). In the words of the parent of one of our panel of dyslexic children, it might be that life for a dyslexic child is like living in a foreign country where one knows the language pretty well, and it is possible to get by adequately, but only at the expense of continual concentration and effort.

This belief in a skill acquisition deficit led us to formulate and test two linked working hypotheses: first, the Dyslexic Automatisation Deficit (DAD) hypothesis, that dyslexic children have unusual difficulty in automatising any skill, whether motor or cognitive, and second, the 'Conscious Compensation' hypothesis, namely that dyslexic children are normally able to overcome their automatisation deficit by means of consciously compensating for it, that is, by trying harder and/or by using strategies to minimise or mask the deficit. In this review we present three extended studies which we believe provide convincing support for this framework.

Before discussing the experiments individually, it is important to state the basis for our selection of subjects. In brief, we wanted to study 'pure' dyslexia, uncontaminated by factors such as low IQ, economic disadvantage, and so on. Consequently, we used the standard exclusionary criterion of 'children of normal or above normal IQ (operationalised as IQ of 90 or more on the Wechsler

Intelligence Scale for Children), without known primary emotional or behavioural or socioeconomic problems, whose reading age (RA) was at least 18 months behind their chronological age (CA).'

Study 2: Balance and automaticity

Our first set of experiments provided a critical test of the DAD/CC hypothesis. We reasoned that there was little point choosing tasks related to reading or language, in that existing empirical data suggested that there should be deficits there. A more rigorous test of the theory was for a skill in which there was thought to be little or no deficit. We decided to test motor skill, and in particular the gross motor skill of balance, on the basis that this was one of the most highly practised of all skills, with absolutely no linguistic involvement. Full details of the study are provided in Nicolson and Fawcett (1990). Our subjects were 23 dyslexic children around 13 years old and 8 normal children, with groups matched overall for age and IQ. We monitored their performance for three tasks, standing on both feet, one in front of the other; standing on one foot; and walking. All three tasks took place on a low 'beam' 4 inches high and 4 inches across, made of large plastic bricks. Balance performance was determined by videotaping each session, with separate cameras for hands and feet, and subsequently scoring each session for wobbles, assigning a half point for a small wobble (10–20°), one point for a medium wobble (20–50°) and two points for a major wobble (overbalancing or putting one foot down). Scoring was independently checked by a scorer blind to the identity of each subject. The balance tasks were performed under two conditions: single task balance, in which the subjects had merely to balance; and dual task balance, in which they had to balance while undertaking a further secondary task. Two secondary tasks were used: either counting or performing a choice reaction task. Each secondary task was initially 'calibrated' so as to be of equivalent difficulty for each subject, by adjusting the task difficulty (for counting) or by providing extended training (for choice reactions) so that, under 'just counting' or 'just choice reaction' conditions all subjects fell into the same performance band. In a further study (Fawcett and Nicolson, 1992), we replicated this study using five groups of dyslexic and control children (with the design as in study

1, using dyslexic children at 11 and 15, together with control groups at 8, 11 and 15 years, thereby allowing both chronological age match and reading age match comparisons).

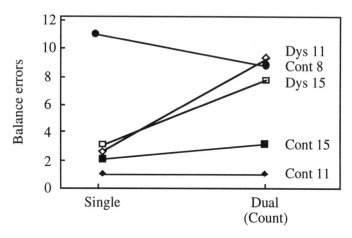

Figure 6.2a Balance results (counting, both feet)

The results for both studies followed exactly the same pattern, and those for Fawcett and Nicolson (1992) are shown in Figure 6.2a. They are exactly as predicted by DAD/CC. Under single task balance conditions there was no difference in balance between the groups. Under dual task conditions the dyslexic children showed a highly significant impairment in balance, whereas the control children showed no deficit. Furthermore, if one considers performance on the dual task, the dyslexic children showed a significant impairment when balancing (as opposed to their performance on the dual task by itself) whereas the normal children showed no such impairment. Even more convincing, in addition to the significant differences at the group level, the pattern of performance also applied to almost all the individuals, with 22 out of the 23 dyslexic children in the original study showing a decrement under dual task conditions whereas most of the controls actually improved (owing, no doubt, to the effect of practice). The individual data for this 'balance impairment' (i.e., the increase in wobbles under dual task conditions compared with normal conditions) for the 1992 study are shown in Figure 6.2b. It may be seen that all the 11-year-old dyslexics and 14 out of 16 of the 15-year-old dyslexics showed a balance impairment, whereas the controls tended not to show any impairment.

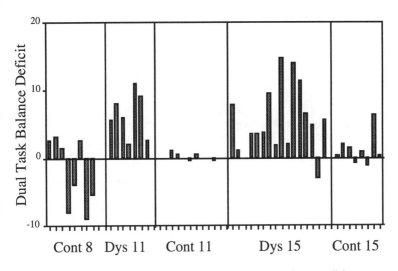

Figure 6.2b Individual balance deficit in the counting condition

One problem with the dual task impairments is that it is not clear whether the impairment is attributable to prevention of conscious compensation (as predicted by DAD) or some more general attentional deficit which causes impairments whenever two tasks must be performed simultaneously. In order to discriminate between these accounts we performed a further series of experiments (Fawcett and Nicolson, 1992) in which we blindfolded the subjects, thereby preventing conscious compensation but not introducing the complications of a dual task paradigm. As predicted, the group of dyslexic children showed much greater impairment than the controls when blindfolded, further support for the DAD/CC hypothesis (Figure 6.3a). The individual results for blindfold balance impairment (Figure 6.3b) are if anything even more striking than those for dual task balance impairments.

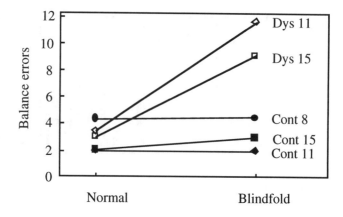

Figure 6.3a Blindfold balance

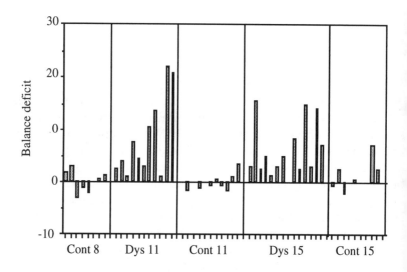

Figure 6.3b Individual balance deficits in two-foot blindfold condition

LONG-TERM LEARNING AND DYSLEXIA

The above studies provide powerful support for the DAD/CC hypothesis, in that a specific, and unexpected, pattern of results was predicted and discovered. Looked at critically, however, the studies provided more support for the concept of conscious compensation than for DAD, in that any theory which predicted a motor skill deficit could provide an account of the pattern of results. The only way to provide direct evidence for or against DAD was to undertake a long-term training study on a novel skill, and to attempt to identify in which stage, if any, the dyslexic children showed impaired performance. Two studies were undertaken, using children from the same group as those used for the initial balance experiments. To our knowledge, these are the only studies of long-term skill acquisition in the dyslexia literature.

Study 3: Becoming fluent at Pacman

The first study involved learning a complex eye–hand coordination skill, typical of everyday activity of many teenage children, namely performance on an arcade-type computer game, specially redesigned to allow performance speed and accuracy to be monitored continuously. The subjects had to navigate the 'Pacman' icon round a fixed track of a computer maze, using specified key presses to move left, right, up and down. The critical question was how the skills developed with practice, and so extended training was given over a period of about 6 months until each subject appeared to have stopped improving. Performance was monitored three times per session at 20-minute intervals, with the intervening time taken up with free play on the full game, together with various other tests as part of our testing program. Following a two-week respite from the task, the key–movement mappings were then changed incompatibly, thereby forcing the subjects to unlearn their initial finger–movement pairings and to relearn the new pairings, and performance was again monitored until no noticeable improvement was taking place. Finally, one year later, the task was administered again, this time with eight fixed sessions of three trials, in order to examine the amount of forgetting of the skill over one year. Furthermore, various perturbations to the standard procedure were made on the later sessions, in order to examine the susceptibility of the skill to interference. Twenty-one subjects participated, with 13 of our original dyslexic group and the original 8 controls. Full details are presented in Nicolson and Fawcett (1993).

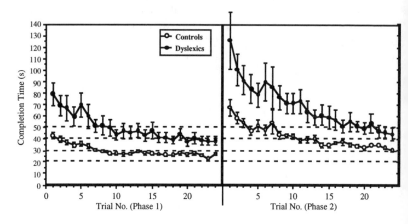

Figure 6.4 Pacman completion times in phases 1 and 2
(error bars are the standard errors)

The results for the completion times for the first two phases are shown in Figure 6.4. The dyslexic children were initially very much slower than the controls, and even after extended training they were still significantly slower. On the other hand, they showed good improvement in speed with practice, and also showed equivalent interference to the controls when the key mappings were changed. Similar results were obtained for errors (incorrect key presses), with the dyslexic children making significantly more errors initially and after training, but in contrast to their completion times, and in contrast to the control children, the dyslexic children showed little reduction in error rate with training.

In order to obtain more accurate estimates of the learning rates for completion times and errors, the group data were fitted using a parametric technique which has been established as the most appropriate for fitting human data on practice (Newell and Rosenbloom, 1981).

In brief, the curve fitted is the 'power law' $P(n) = A + Bn^{-\alpha}$ where $P(n)$ refers to performance on trial n, A is the asymptotic performance as $n \to \infty$, B is a scaling parameter linked directly to initial performance, and α is the learning rate. The best fit was derived by a least squares technique, though the details are beyond the scope of this chapter. For phase 1 the equations for completion time were $T = 20 + 92.0 \ n^{-0.51}$ for the dyslexic children and $T = 20 + 33.7 \ n^{-0.59}$ for the controls. In neither Phase 1 nor 2 was there a significant difference in learning rate, and the major difference was in the parameter B, initial performance. By contrast, the learning rate for error elimination was markedly lower for the dyslexic children, to the extent that the model predicts that the dyslexic children would be making more errors after 10,000 trials than the normal children after 100 trials! For phase 1 the corresponding models for error rate E were $E = 26.1 \ n^{-0.11}$ for the dyslexic children and $E = 21.9 \ n^{-0.22}$ for the controls. Performance in phase 3 indicated that both groups showed good skill retention over the intervening year, and also good relearning, in that after only two sessions of three trials both groups were performing around the level of their previous best performance. Furthermore, the dyslexic children appeared to be able to cope as well as the controls with changes of layout, with presentation of white noise, and with the need to undertake an auditory detection task while navigating round the maze. Fuller descriptions are provided in Nicolson and Fawcett (1993).

We concluded from this study that, under these near-optimal conditions for the development of automatisation, the dyslexic children had a normal 'strength' of automatisation, as evidenced by difficulty of unlearning, by retention over one year, and by resistance to interfering tasks, but that they showed a lower 'quality' of automatised performance, in terms both of speed and accuracy. Learning rate showed some dissociation, with normal rate of improvement in speed, but impaired rate of improvement in accuracy. Over and above these differences in learning parameters, however, was the marked difference in initial performance, presumably reflecting difficulties in proceduralising the task, since the declarative nature of the task is very simple.

Interesting though these results are, their theoretical interpretation is clouded by the fact that the task was actually quite close to several real world tasks. It may be, for instance, that the results underestimate the potential of the dyslexic children, with part of their initial performance deficits being attributable to the well-known problems dyslexic children have discriminating right from left (Miles, 1983), or maybe to a comparative lack of prior practice on some of the component skills. On the other hand, it may be that these results overestimate the learning potential of the dyslexic children. Perhaps their near-normal rate of improvement in speed is partly attributable to the fact that they had much more room for improvement than the control children. These issues could only be resolved by a further experiment, one in which we attempted to ensure that the dyslexic children had no impairment on the component skills underlying the task to be learned.

Study 4: Blending of subskills into a complex skill

In related research (Nicolson and Fawcett, 1994; see study 1), we had established that this group of dyslexic children had normal speed of simple reaction (that is, pressing a button as soon as they heard a low tone), but that their speed of choice reaction was impaired compared with same age controls. Interestingly, this impairment obtained even to a selective choice reaction, in which the target tone and the response was identical to that of the simple reaction, but an alternative low tone was presented on half the trials for which the subject had to make no response. With the intention of further probing this intriguing dissociation, while studying the time course of the automatisation process for a primitive skill, we conducted a further long-term training study, in which we examined the time course of development of choice reaction speed. In order to avoid any problems of left–right confusions or of stimulus discriminability, we used two stimuli of different modalities (tone and flash) and different effectors (hand and foot) for the two stimuli. Twenty-two subjects participated, 11 dyslexic and 11 control, with the bulk of them being the tireless participants in the earlier studies. In brief, following baseline performance monitoring on simple reaction to each stimulus separately (counterbalanced so that half the subjects had the hand-button paired with the tone, and the foot-button paired with the flash, and the other half vice versa), the two simple reaction tasks were combined into a choice reaction task in which half the stimuli were tones and half flashes, and the subject had to press the corresponding button, using the mapping established in the simple reactions. Each session comprised three runs, each of 100 stimuli, and as in the previous study subjects kept returning every fortnight or so until their performance stopped improving (in terms of speed and accuracy). The results are shown in Figure 6.5.

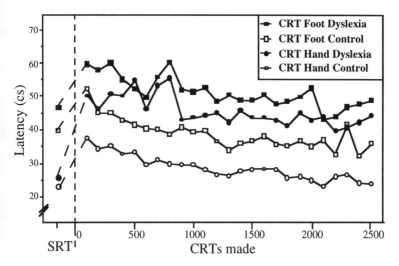

Figure 6.5 Median latencies over the period of CRT training

Analysis of the simple reaction performance indicated that there were no significant differences between the groups either for foot or hand, tone or flash. By contrast, initial performance on the choice reaction was significantly slower, and final performance was both significantly slower and less accurate for the dyslexic children. A parametric learning rate analysis was then performed using the power law equation outlined above. The best fit curves for hand response CRT were $t = 53.9 \, n^{-0.073}$ for the dyslexic children and $t = 39.4 \, n^{-0.141}$ for the controls. For the foot responses the corresponding best fit curves were $t = 62.3 \, n^{-0.086}$; $t = 50.4 \, n^{-0.116}$ respectively. As in the Pacman experiment, the parameter B was higher for the dyslexic children than the controls (around 30% on average). This is a particularly interesting result in view of the near-equality of the baseline simple reaction performance on which the CRT was founded. Even more interesting, however, is the difference in learning rate in this experiment. It may be seen that α is twice as large for the controls than the dyslexic children for manual responses (0.141 vs. 0.073) and one third larger for the foot responses (0.116 vs. 0.086). This is a huge difference. Bearing in mind that the learning varies as a function of the time to the power α, if a skill takes a normal child 100 hours to master, it would, taking an average ratio of the learning rates as say 1.5, take a dyslexic child $100^{1.5}$ i.e. 1,000 hours (10 times as long) to learn the skill to the same criterion.

The availability of data from training on two quite different skills strengthens the possible interpretation of the results. In particular, it seems reasonable to ascribe the initial performance decrement found in both experiments to a real difficulty in the initial proceduralisation of skill. Furthermore lower 'quality' of automatisation (indexed by speed and by errors) was found in both studies. It seems reasonable, therefore, to argue that this group of dyslexic children have difficulties with the initial proceduralisation of skill, and with the 'quality' of skill post-training, but that the 'strength' of skill automatisation is normal. The rate of improvement with practice (α) appeared normal in the Pacman study but was markedly impaired in the CRT training study. If the CRT training results apply to dyslexic children generally, and apply to tasks other than choice reactions, we are led to a radically new prediction for dyslexic performance, namely that rather than being at the level of children of their own age, or even, as is often considered the appropriate control group, children of the same reading age, the performance of dyslexic children on any task will be comparable with that of much younger children, with the amount of impairment increasing as the square root of the necessary learning time.

OVERALL DISCUSSION

In this chapter we have covered a good deal of ground, reviewing research on speed of processing and on motor skills, and presenting studies on speed of processing, balance and skill acquisition. The speed of processing study revealed difficulties in choice reactions, even with non-linguistic material, and even though speed of simple reaction was normal. Performance on choice reactions was at the level of the reading age controls. The tests of balance revealed that the apparently normal balance performance of the dyslexic children masked an underlying deficit (normally concealed via conscious attentional compensation), in that performance in dual task circumstances or when blindfolded was at a lower level even than reading age controls. We interpreted this as reflecting incomplete automatisation of the balance skill. The tests of long-term skill acquisition suggested that dyslexic children were able to automatise skills, but that even when automatised, performance was at a lower level than normal (in terms of speed and accuracy). Somewhat different findings as to learning rate emerged, in that the dyslexic children showed near-normal speed of acquisition of the hand–eye coordination Pacman skills, whereas their learning rate appeared to be significantly impaired in the speed of processing choice reaction task. A common finding to both acquisition studies was the very poor initial performance.

There are direct parallels between the studies reported in this chapter and issues raised in other chapters. Most directly relevant is the link between this work and the findings of reduced automaticity and greater need for conscious compensation in reading identified by Yap and van der Leij (Chapter 3). The issue of speed of processing has recurred throughout the book (Chapters 3, 4 and 5) and it is by no means resolved here. Indeed, it may be that the apparently greater difficulty in learning the choice reaction task as opposed to the hand–eye task does reflect some rather intractable difficulties in speeded information processing. Whilst our acquisition studies did not investigate the processes of reading, they would appear to support the findings of Yap and van der Leij that there will be difficulties in speeded reading, whereas other aspects should be acquired relatively normally (after a delayed start), thereby addressing the issue of intractability raised by Beech.

We conclude this chapter with an analysis of the automatisation deficit/conscious compensation hypothesis, taking as our task an evaluation of the hypothesis using the four criteria stated by Rack (chapter 1), namely *specificity* (why does the problem appear to be specific to reading-related skills rather than more general cognitive abilities?), *causality* (are automatisation deficits the cause, a consequence or a correlate of the reading problems?), *process* (can one specify the process by which automatisation deficits result in reading problems?) and *variation* (are differences in severity of automatisation deficit sufficient to account for individual variations in reading difficulty?).

The explanation is in fact markedly different from that put forward by phonological deficit theorists, especially with respect to specificity. Rather than accepting that the skill deficits are specific to reading-related skills, we propose, on the contrary, that the reading-related deficits are merely the tip of an iceberg, and that almost all primitive skills (such as speed of processing and motor skill) are likely to be impaired. The reason, we argue, for the apparent specificity of skill deficits is that dyslexic children succeed in masking the deficit for many skills and for many situations, consciously compensating for their incomplete automatisation by trying harder. The identification of hitherto unsuspected deficits both in choice reactions to non-linguistic stimuli (study 1) and in the gross motor skill of balance (study 2) provide striking support for the hypothesis that dyslexic children are impaired in even the most basic skills.

Deficits will be apparent in situations where conscious compensation is not possible. These situations include: complex skills (such as reading) which require fluency in the component subskills; time-dependent skills in which processing speed is at a premium; dual tasks (such as remembering what to do while walking upstairs) and multi-modality skills (such as soccer) where it is necessary to monitor several modalities or information sources simultaneously; and also vigilance situations, where tiredness will occur more rapidly and also have more severe effects upon performance. By contrast, dyslexic athletes might excel at 'closed' sports such as swimming and track athletics, where it is possible (and even desirable) to concentrate purely on one's own actions, and not be distracted by information from other sources.

An important issue related to specificity is that raised by several colleagues: assuming that dyslexic children suffer from a general problem in skill acquisition, how do they ever become proficient in any aspect of their lives? Why are they not just useless at everything? It is here that the skill acquisition studies (study 3 and 4, this chapter) are valuable. Note, first, that in both studies the dyslexic children showed impaired skill initially, but that they learned reasonably well (in the Pacman study the learning was actually faster than the controls), and they were able to automatise the skills (though performance quality was lower). Note, second, that the dyslexic children had equivalent IQ (as measured by the WISC) to the control groups. Although there are problems with skill, their basic cognitive apparatus is functioning well. They will be able to adapt, think creatively, notice relevant facts, and show flexibility in behaviour (indeed, if one is used to using one's mind to compensate for deficiencies in one's skills, it may well be that this leads to considerably better use of the mental resources available). Over and above these cognitive factors, it is very likely that motivational factors hold the key to success in later life. Anyone who has seen a successful dyslexic at work will appreciate the value of refusing to be beaten and the burning determination to prove wrong those teachers who had labelled them as stupid.

Let us now turn to causality. We believe that the automatisation deficits cause the reading problems by two related routes. First, reading is one of the most complex skills which children are routinely required to master, demanding the smooth interplay of a range of subskills for expert performance (LaBerge and Samuels, 1974), and deficits in even one of these skills can lead to impaired performance. Therefore reading acts as a litmus test for any skill problems. If the low-level components of reading, such as letter recognition and grapheme–phoneme translation, continue to demand conscious attention, the attentional resources required to undertake the next stage, phoneme blending into syllables and then into words, are no longer available, and progress will not be made. Second, the DAD/CC predicts that dyslexic children will typically show phonological deficits, in that phonological skills are learned, and one would therefore assume dyslexic children would require greater attentional resources to acquire them. Whenever there is time stress on phonological skills, one would expect dyslexic children to show deficits. Consequently, one might see the phonological deficit hypothesis as subsumed by our more general automatisation deficit hypothesis, and the causal links between phonological skill deficits and reading deficits described by Rack can apply equally to the automatisation deficit hypothesis, with the added point that the latter also gives a reasonable account of why speed of processing proves to be less tractable than other aspects of reading for dyslexic children.

Consider next, process. The general account provided by automatisation deficit theory is essentially that given above. Skill acquisition difficulties lead to reduced phonological skills, together with the need for greater conscious involvement. These two difficulties combine to cause severe reading problems which, though not completely intractable (see studies 3 and 4) require the input of a great deal more time and effort than normal, and probably call for a much more systematic approach to teaching the basic reading subskills.

The final issue, that of individual differences, has not been discussed here. Whilst it is quite possible that the strength of automatisation deficit will correlate strongly with the reading deficit, the studies described in this chapter are not sufficient to assess the case. Such an investigation requires the collection of information on a range of skills for each child, and then a correlational analysis. We address this issue in our final chapter. For the time being, it is encouraging to note that almost all of the dyslexic children in our studies have in fact also shown the impairment in balance under dual task or blindfold conditions.

In conclusion, in this chapter we have considered performance of dyslexic children on a range of skills including speed of processing, motor skill and balance. There is no doubt that there are clear signs of deficit in most of these skills, especially when the child is not allowed to consciously compensate for deficits in the skill in question. Our proposal that dyslexic children suffer from deficits in skill automatisation gives an excellent general account of the range of deficits shown. There remains suggestive evidence (echoing suggestions made by many of the contributors to this volume) that deficits in speeded processing are rather less tractable than others. However, it should be stressed that labelling the deficit as one of automatisation does not explain which aspect(s) of the automatisation process are impaired or why. Search for the mechanism underlying these deficits is a task for further research, and one which we address in the final chapter.

REFERENCES

Adams, M.J. (1990). *Beginning to Read: Thinking and learning about print.* Cambridge, MA: MIT Press.

Anderson, J.R. (1982). Acquisition of cognitive skill. *Psychological Review, 89,* 369–406.

Anderson, J.R. (1989). A theory of the origins of human knowledge. *Artificial Intelligence, 40,* 313–351.

Augur, J. (1985). Guidelines for teachers, parents and learners. In M. Snowling (Ed.), *Children's Written Language Difficulties* (pp. 147–171). Windsor, UK: NFER Nelson.

Benton, A.L. (1978). Some conclusions about dyslexia. In A.L. Benton and D. Pearl (Eds.), *Dyslexia: An appraisal of current knowledge.* New York: Oxford University Press.

Bowers, P.G., Steffy, R.A. and Tate, E. (1988). Comparison of the effects of IQ control methods on memory and naming speed predictors of reading disability. *Reading Research Quarterly, 23,* 304–319.

Bradley, L. (1988). Making connections in learning to read and to spell. *Applied Cognitive Psychology, 2,* 3–18.

Bradley, L. and Bryant, P.E. (1983). Categorising sounds and learning to read: A causal connection. *Nature, 301,* 419–421.

Brady, S., Shankweiler, D. and Mann, V. (1983). Speech perception and memory coding in relation to naming ability. *Journal of Experimental Child Psychology, 35,* 345–367.

Bryant, P. and Goswami, U. (1986). Strengths and weaknesses of the reading level design. *Psychological Bulletin, 100,* 101–103.

Catts, H.W. (1986). Speech production/phonological deficits in developmental dyslexia. *Journal of Learning Disabilities, 19,* 504–508.

Catts, H.W. (1989). Defining dyslexia as a developmental language disorder. *Annals of Dyslexia, 39,* 50–64.

Coles, M.G.H., Gratton, G. and Fabiani, M. (1990). Event related brain potentials. In J.T. Cacioppo and L.G. Tassinary (Eds.), *Principles of Psychophysiology: Physical, social and inferential elements.* Cambridge: Cambridge University Press.

Denckla, M.B. (1985). Motor co-ordination in dyslexic children: Theoretical and clinical implications. In F.H. Duffy and N. Geschwind (Eds.), *Dyslexia: A neuroscientific approach to clinical evaluation.* Boston, MA: Little, Brown.

Denckla, M.B. and Rudel, R.G. (1976). Rapid 'Automatised' naming (R.A.N.): Dyslexia differentiated from other learning disabilities. *Neuropsychologia, 14,* 471–479.

Donders, F.C. (1868). Over de snelheid van psychische processen: Onder-zoekingen gedaan in het Psychologish Laboratorium der Utrechtsche Hoogeschool: 1868–69. Tweede Reeks, II, 92–120. (trans. W.G. Koster) *Attention and Performance II. Acta Psychologica,* 1969, *30,* 412–431.

Ellis, N.C. and Miles, T.R. (1981). A lexical encoding difficulty I: Experimental evidence. In G.Th. Pavlidis and T.R. Miles (Eds.), *Dyslexia Research and its Application to Education.* Chichester: Wiley.

Fawcett, A.J. (1990) *A Cognitive Architecture of Dyslexia.* Unpublished PhD thesis, University of Sheffield, UK.

Fawcett, A.J. and Nicolson, R.I. (1992). Automatisation deficits in balance for dyslexic children. *Perceptual and Motor Skills, 75,* 507–529.

Fawcett, A.J., Chattopadhyay, A.K., Kandler, R.H., Jarratt, J.A., Nicolson, R.I. and Proctor, M. (1993). Event-related potentials and dyslexia. *Annals of the New York Academy of Sciences, 682,* 342–345.

Felton, R.H., Wood, F.B., Brown, I.S. and Campbell, S.K. (1987). Separate verbal memory and naming deficits in attention deficit disorder and reading disability. *Brain and Language, 31,* 171–184.

Fitts, P.M. and Posner, M.I. (1967). *Human Performance.* Belmont, CA: Brooks Cole.

Gathercole, S.E. and Baddeley, A.D. (1990). Phonological memory deficits in language disordered children: Is there a causal connection? *Journal of Memory and Language, 29,* 336–360.

Haslum, M.N. (1989). Predictors of dyslexia? *Irish Journal of Psychology, 10,* 622–630.

Hulme, C., Maughan, S. and Brown, G.D.A. (1991). Memory for familiar and unfamiliar words: Evidence for a long-term memory contribution to short-term memory span. *Journal of Memory and Language, 30,* 685–701.

LaBerge, D. and Samuels, S.J. (1974). Toward a theory of automatic information processing in reading. *Cognitive Psychology, 6,* 293–323.

Livingstone, M.S., Rosen, G.D., Drislane, F.W. and Galaburda, A.M. (1991). Physiological and anatomical evidence for a magnocellular defect in developmental dyslexia. *Proceedings of the National Academy of Sciences of the USA, 88,* 7943–7947.

Lundberg, I. and Høien, T. (1989). Phonemic deficits: A core symptom of developmental dyslexia? *Irish Journal of Psychology, 10,* 579–592.

Miles, T.R. (1983). *Dyslexia: The pattern of difficulties.* Blackwell: Oxford.

Miles, T.R. (1993). *Dyslexia: The pattern of difficulties* (2nd edition). London: Whurr.

Miles, T.R. and Miles, E. (1990). *Dyslexia: A hundred years on.* Milton Keynes: Open University Press.

Newell, A. and Rosenbloom, P.S. (1981). Mechanisms of skill acquisition and the law of practice. In J.R. Anderson (Ed.), *Cognitive Skills and their Acquisition.* Hillsdale, NJ: Lawrence Erlbaum.

Newton, M.J. and Thomson, M.E. (1976). *The Aston Index.* Wisbech, Cambridge: Learning Development Aids.

Nicolson, R.I. and Fawcett, A.J. (1990). Automaticity: A new framework for dyslexia research? *Cognition, 35,* 159–182.

Nicolson, R.I. (1982). Cognitive factors in simple reactions: A developmental study. *Journal of Motor Behavior, 14,* 69–80.

Nicolson, R.I. and Fawcett, A.J. (1993). Children with dyslexia automatise temporal skills more slowly. *Annals of the New York Academy of Sciences, 682,* 390–392.

Nicolson, R.I. and Fawcett, A.J. (1994). Reaction times and dyslexia. *Quarterly Journal of Experimental Psychology, 47A,* 1–16.

Olson, R.K., Wise, B.W. and Rack, J.P. (1989). Dyslexia: Deficits, genetic aetiology and computer based remediation. *Irish Journal of Psychology, 10,* 594–608.

Rudel, R.G. (1985). The definition of dyslexia: Language and motor deficits. In F.H. Duffy and N. Geschwind (Eds.), *Dyslexia: A neuroscientific approach to clinical evaluation* (pp. 33–53). Boston, MA: Little, Brown.

Rudel, R.G., Denckla, M.B. and Broman, M. (1981). The effect of varying stimulus context on word finding ability: Dyslexia further differentiated from other reading disabilities. *Brain and Language, 13,* 130–144.

Seymour, P.H.K. (1986). *Cognitive Analysis of Dyslexia.* London: Routledge and Kegan Paul.

Shiffrin, R.M., Dumais, S.T. and Schneider, W. (1981). Characteristics of automatism. In J. Long and A.D. Baddeley (Eds.), *Attention and Performance IX* (pp. 223–238). London: Lawrence Erlbaum.

Shiffrin, R.M. and Schneider, W. (1977). Controlled and automatic human information processing: II. Perceptual learning, automatic attending and general theory. *Psychological Review, 84,* 127–190.

Snowling, M.J. (1981). Phonemic deficits in developmental dyslexia. *Psychological Research, 43,* 219–234.

Snowling, M.J., Goulandris, N., Bowlby, M. and Howell, P. (1986). Segmentation and speech perception in relation to reading skill: A developmental analysis. *Journal of Experimental Child Psychology, 41,* 489–507.

Stanovich, K.E. (1986). Matthew effects in reading: Some consequences of individual differences in the acquisition of literacy. *Reading Research Quarterly, 21,* 360–407.

Stanovich, K.E. (1988). The right and wrong places to look for the cognitive locus of reading disability. *Annals of Dyslexia, 38,* 154–177.

Swanson, H.L. (1987). Verbal coding deficits in the recall of pictorial information by learning disabled readers: The influence of a lexical system. *American Educational Research Journal, 24,* 143–170.

Tallal, P. (1980). Auditory temporal perception, phonics and reading disability in children. *Brain and Language, 9*, 182–198.

Tallal, P. (1983). Acoustic coding of speech and normal limits on transfer of information: A discussion paper. *Annals of the New York Academy of Science, 405*, 64–65.

Tallal, P. and Stark, R.E. (1982). Perceptual/motor profiles of reading impaired children with or without concomitant oral language deficits. *Annals of Dyslexia, 32*, 163–176.

Tallal, P., Stark, R.E. and Mellits, D. (1985). The relationship between auditory temporal analysis and receptive language development: Evidence from studies of developmental language disorder. *Neuropsychologia, 23*, 527–534.

Thomson, M.E. (1991). The teaching of spelling using techniques of simultaneous oral spelling and visual inspection. In M. Snowling and M. Thomson (Eds.), *Dyslexia: Integrating theory and practice.* London: Whurr.

Tomblin, J.B. and Quinn, M.A. (1983). The contribution of perceptual learning to performance on the repetition task. *Journal of Speech and Hearing Research, 26*, 369–372.

Urion, D.K., Wolf, M., Kleinman, S.N. and Kilcoyne Young, P. (1987). Patterns of neurological, reading and language functions among dyslexic and average readers. Report, Child Study Department, Tufts University, Massachusetts.

Vellutino, F.R. (1979). *Dyslexia: Theory and research.* Cambridge, MA: MIT Press.

Wechsler, D. (1976). *Wechsler Intelligence Scale for Children (WISC–R).* Slough: NFER.

Wolf, M. (1991). Naming speed and reading: The contribution of the cognitive neurosciences. *Reading Research Quarterly, 26*, 123–141.

Wolf, M. and Obregon, M. (1992). Early naming deficits, developmental dyslexia, and a specific deficit hypothesis. *Brain and Language, 42*, 219–247.

Wolff, P.H., Cohen, C. and Drake, C. (1984). Impaired motor timing control in specific reading retardation. *Neuropsychologia, 22*, 587–600.

Wolff, P.H., Michel, G.F. and Ovrut, M. (1990a). Rate variables and automatised naming in developmental dyslexia. *Brain and Language, 39*, 556–575.

Wolff, P.H., Michel, G.F. and Ovrut, M. (1990b). Rate and timing precision of motor co-ordination in developmental dyslexia. *Developmental Psychology, 26*, 349–359.

Wolff, P.H., Michel, G.F. and Ovrut, M. (1990c). The timing of syllable repetitions in developmental dyslexia. *Journal of Speech and Hearing Research, 33*, 281–289.

PART 3

Towards the underlying causes of dyslexia

The reviews in the previous two parts have presented summaries of large bodies of data, with each chapter focusing on a different skill or set of skills. One might see Parts 1 and 2 as approaches to analysing the performance characteristics of dyslexic children into their various different components. In this final part, we wished to attempt the converse operation, taking the specific deficits identified in the earlier chapters, and trying to piece them together in the hope of finding some coherent pattern, or even some approach to finding a coherent underlying pattern.

Consequently, we felt it appropriate at this stage to provide a chapter from Tim Miles on the issues involved in diagnosing dyslexia, with particular reference to the question of how to cope with the problem that dyslexic children appear to be very heterogeneous, each showing a different constellation of difficulties. He is, of course, particularly well placed to provide this overview, having extensive experience of diagnosis of dyslexia, and in particular having developed the Bangor Dyslexia Test, the first test to provide positive indicators of dyslexia rather than rely on discrepancy scores.

In this chapter, having had an opportunity to read the earlier chapters, Professor Miles puts forward the concept of a 'taxonomy' – a principled system of classification – as applied to dyslexia which must be able to accommodate the different characterisations of dyslexia that occur in this book. He suggests that whether you decide to 'lump' dyslexic children together or 'split' them into different groups depends on your objectives: it may be appropriate to consider dyslexic children as a heterogeneous group (lumping) for the purpose of hypothesis testing, while recognising the need to consider their heterogeneity (splitting) in order to measure individual differences. Using the analogy of splitting rock, he argues that, although there are a variety of ways in which the rock may be split, some are more fruitful than others in producing a meaningful chunk rather than disconnected fragments. It is important that a taxonomy be proposed from a position of knowledge if we are to produce a strong taxonomy, that is one which leads to theories of wide generality.

Following a historical overview of the concept of taxonomy in relation to the biological sciences, Miles presents the characteristics of the proposed taxonomy. He suggests that the taxonomy must be capable of recognising the links between seven different areas; anatomical and genetic findings; postulated deficits in the magnocellular and transient systems, and in impaired auditory processing speed; an identifiable pattern of difficulties noted in the biographical studies; and phonological deficits. Inclusion of these areas allows dyslexia to become a more powerful concept than simply poor reading. In fact, overemphasis on reading diverts attention away from the other difficulties experienced by dyslexics, in particular their slowness in processing. Diagnosis by exclusion is criticised because it lacks positive indicators which persist over time, in favour of reading deficits which are more amenable to remediation. It is argued that we should be concerned with the imbalance of skills in the dyslexic population, rather than the traditional interpretation of the IQ test. Professor Miles concludes that those who show this imbalance between phonological and reasoning skills may rightly be lumped together as dyslexic, and equally those who simply show poor reading should continue to be split.

Finally, for reasons which may be substantially attributed to the editors, there has been some delay between the time the majority of these chapters was written and the time the book was finally completed. This has given us the opportunity to write a final chapter including the results of some of our recent work which addresses directly the issues raised by Miles, and gives, for the first time, a comprehensive survey of the abilities of dyslexic children across the range of primitive skills. The research design facilitates comparison of the depth of deficit of the various skills, while also providing an estimate of the incidence of significant deficits in each subject for each skill. Dyslexic children (mean ages 8, 13 and 17 years), control groups of normally achieving children matched for IQ and for age or reading age, and 'slow learner' children matched for reading age with the youngest dyslexic children, were tested on a range of primitive skills. The dyslexic children performed significantly worse than the same-age controls on most tasks, and significantly worse even than the reading age controls on segmentation, picture naming speed, temporal estimation and blindfold balance. The slow learners had significantly better balance and significantly worse phonological skill and processing speed than the matched dyslexic group. Individual analyses found no evidence of subtypes of dyslexia, in that almost all the dyslexic children showed the pattern of impaired phonological skill and impaired balance.

Whilst the overall performance of the dyslexic children may be characterised as showing less complete automatisation than normal, none of the existing theories of dyslexia provides a convincing account of the specific pattern of deficits, and their changes with age. In a final, more speculative, analysis, we present evidence that the specific pattern of deficits is consistent with early cerebellar damage, demonstrating that the hypothesis generates novel predictions which were confirmed by an empirical test. In conclusion, we argue that cerebellar deficit forms the basis for the 'strong taxonomy' advocated by Miles. We hope that further research will lead to the emergence of new taxonomies.

CHAPTER 7

A proposed taxonomy and some consequences

T. R. Miles

INTRODUCTION

The central theme of this chapter is the concept of 'taxonomy'. It will be suggested that different characterisations of dyslexia – such as those that occur in this book – can usefully be regarded as proposals for different taxonomies. The implications of one particular taxonomy will then be explored.

When people disagree as to where to draw boundaries they are aligning themselves, whether explicitly or implicitly, with either 'lumpers' or 'splitters' – lumpers being those who wish to group certain things together, and splitters those who wish to emphasise their separateness. That this is a problem in the classification of language disorders was recognised by Denckla (1972), but since that date the idea does not seem to have been explicitly taken up.

There is no special merit in either lumping or splitting as such. Hypothesis building may require us to lump together phenomena which seemed *prima facie* unconnected, and this can sometimes constitute a significant advance; on the other hand, as knowledge increases and researchers become more sensitive to differences there may be increased pressures towards splitting. Whether one should be a lumper or a splitter will therefore depend on the circumstances of a particular case.

Once this point is recognised the way becomes open for some of the apparent conflicts in disputed areas to be resolved: both parties may be right, since lumping may be appropriate for one purpose and splitting for another. Moreover, since boundaries often need to be changed as science advances, there is no need to fan the flames of controversy by insisting that a particular boundary is the only correct one to draw.

However, this does not justify a *laissez faire* attitude towards the selection of a taxonomy. As will be seen in a moment, some taxonomies are 'stronger' (or more powerful) than others; and if one's objective is scientific research it is inefficient to use a weaker taxonomy when a stronger one is available. The following analogy (which I owe to Dr Rod Nicolson) may be of help in this connection. There are all kinds of places where one might apply pressure to a rock; but if one applies pressure exactly along a fault line the resultant division of the rock will provide meaningful 'chunks' for further study. In contrast, if one applies pressure in other places one will be confronted merely with a collection of disconnected fragments, and it will be difficult to make sense of them. Using this analogy, one might say that the present chapter is an attempt to explore one particular fault line and to work out the implications of doing so.

There is a further reason why some taxonomies can be better than others. If a taxonomy is proposed from a position of strength – from a position of knowledge – then a particular decision to lump or split merits nothing but respect. If two researchers are both aware of all the reasons for lumping and of all the reasons for splitting, then even if one decides to be a lumper and the other a splitter there is nothing significant left for them to disagree about. However, if proposals for classification show lack of such awareness they can justifiably be faulted; and such proposals, regrettably, are not unknown among researchers into reading and literacy.

This chapter will contain an introductory section on taxonomies in general. This will be followed by an indication of some of the important phenomena which require to be grouped together. In the final section there will be a discussion of some of the implications of the proposed taxonomy for teaching and research.

THE CONCEPT OF TAXONOMY

Although the word 'taxonomy' is used primarily by biologists, it would appear that this is largely a matter of historical accident (Heslop-Harrison, 1963, p. 1). What is important for present purposes is to indicate the need for an explicit distinction between what may be called 'strong' and 'weak' taxonomies. In brief, a 'strong' taxonomy is one which leads to theories of wide generality, while a 'weak' taxonomy is one which is valid for limited purposes but which does not point the way to any major advance in scientific knowledge. The distinction between the two can be illustrated by a series of examples.

Let us suppose, in the first place, that the organiser of a conference needs to distinguish those who intend to go on an excursion and those who do not. There is, of course, nothing wrong with such a classification. On the other hand, no one would be tempted to say it was a powerful or strong one; rather it is a classification made for a strictly limited purpose without any implication that it is of any lasting value. In particular there is no suggestion that biological markers – neurological or biochemical differences, for instance – will be discovered which differentiate excursion-goers from non-excursion-goers; nor would one expect biologists to classify them as 'two distinct species' or claim that the distinction heralded a significant scientific breakthrough. In practice the word 'taxonomy' is not used of cases of this kind; but if it were one would have to speak of an extremely weak taxonomy.

It would also be a manifestation of a weak taxonomy if someone were to classify a whale as a fish on the grounds that it lived in the sea or a duck-billed platypus as a bird because it possessed a beak. In both cases it is known that there are a large number of anatomical features which point, beyond doubt, to the classification 'mammal'.

Medicine constitutes an interesting example because some of its taxonomies are very much stronger than others. For example, the terms 'fever' and 'nervous breakdown' still survive in common use since neither is wholly uninformative; if, however, they are contrasted with terms such as 'tuberculosis' and 'phenylketonuria' the differences are plain. It is characteristic of strong medical taxonomies that they imply a theory of causation, accurate prognosis, and distinctive methods of treatment.

The word 'syndrome' is interesting in this connection. *Butterworth's Medical Dictionary* (Critchley, 1978, p. 1647) defines a syndrome as 'a distinct group of symptoms or signs which, associated together, form a characteristic clinical picture or entity'. Similarly *Churchill's Medical Dictionary* (Koenigsberg, 1989, p. 1838) refers to 'signs, symptoms, or other manifestations' and adds that the word is 'used especially when the cause of the condition is unknown'. One can therefore say that use of the term 'syndrome' implies *partial* knowledge; it indicates that we are in possession of a taxonomy of moderate strength even though much more remains to be discovered. This appears to be the present position with regard to dyslexia. If it is agreed that the taxonomy proposed in this chapter has a moderate degree of strength there is in that case every reason for following the lead of Critchley (1981) and others in speaking of dyslexia as a 'syndrome'.

To illustrate further the concept of taxonomy it may be useful at this point to examine how taxonomies develop in other disciplines. The following example from chemistry, which I owe to my friend Dr D.H. Malan, illustrates in a very interesting way how attempts at classification which were not at the time thought to have any special taxonomic power were afterwards recognised as being extremely valuable. It relates to the periodic table of the chemical elements. Dr Malan writes as follows:

> The history of this fundamental concept in chemistry (sc. the periodic table) illustrates the various stages of the development of a taxonomy with great clarity. By the mid-19th century about 70 chemical elements had been discovered, and it began to be noticed that there was some relation between the properties of the elements and their atomic weights. An English chemist, Newlands, found that if elements were arranged in ascending order of atomic weights, then each eighth element resembled the element eight places before it – like octaves in music. But atomic weights were not known accurately enough for this to carry much conviction, and thus Newlands' taxonomy was very weak. Because of this, he was even ridiculed by a member of a learned society, who suggested it would be better to arrange the elements in alphabetical order – which, even more than the 'excursion' taxonomy mentioned above, would be a very weak taxonomy indeed!
>
> Then in the 1860s the Russian chemist Mendeleyev studied the relation between the properties of elements and their atomic weights in great depth,

and came up with a pattern of amazing regularity and equally amazing complexity – which still failed to carry full conviction both because it was so complex and because in many places he had to 'cheat', for instance by leaving gaps in order to complete the pattern. Yet we would now say that the likelihood of the pattern's being due to chance was infinitesimal, and that it was really a taxonomy of great strength – though, since it was constructed retrospectively, no 'significance level' could possibly be calculated. At the same time it lacked the ultimate strength because there was no theoretical basis for it whatsoever. But Mendeleyev had sufficient confidence in his observations to predict that where there were gaps in his pattern new elements would be discovered, and indeed he predicted their properties. Full conviction came when his predictions were repeatedly and almost exactly fulfilled. His taxonomy then became very strong indeed, but it still suffered from the fundamental weakness of lacking any theoretical basis. Nowadays the whole pattern is understood in terms of atomic structure, so that the theoretical basis is firm and conclusive. This is as strong as any taxonomy can possibly be.

In the biological sciences there is similarly a continual search for improved taxonomies. I owe the following account of botanical classification to my colleague, Dr A.J.E. Smith:

> The ancient Greeks classified plants into trees, shrubs, and herbs; these were subdivided into medicinal, agricultural, and other. Linnaeus proposed a classification on the basis of the number of sexual parts to a flower. In contrast phylogenetic classification is based on evolutionary relationships....Taxonomy is very often a matter of opinion and whether one is a lumper or a splitter depends upon one's viewpoint. Usually intimate knowledge leads to splitting, inadequate knowledge to lumping. An example of this is provided by a group of species in the moss genus Fissidens. In Europe, where there have been numerous taxonomists who have carefully studied these plants over the last 150 years, we recognise seven species, five of which can be identified easily in the field. In North America, where expertise is only recent and limited, they recognise only one species saying that it is impossible to discriminate further taxa.

In this case a policy of splitting is being commended on the basis of a claim to greater knowledge, and it is part of the progress of science that such claims to knowledge are continually being tested.

Demarcation of a taxonomy can be achieved either by coining a new word or by making stipulations about the more precise use of a current one. As the word 'dyslexia' lies ready to hand it is the latter policy which will be adopted in this chapter.

CHARACTERISTICS OF THE PROPOSED
TAXONOMY

The following are some of the research findings which require to be lumped together.

(1) It is now widely agreed that the anatomical findings of Albert Galaburda and his colleagues mark a significant advance in knowledge (see in particular Galaburda *et al.*, 1987; Galaburda *et al.*, 1989; Sherman, Rosen and Galaburda, 1989). When *post mortem* examinations were carried out on the brains of eight individuals known to have been dyslexic in their lifetime, it was found in all eight cases that there were structural anomalies (ectopias and dysplasias) and that the two plana were symmetrical (instead of the asymmetry which is reportedly found in 70–80% of cases). Now it is widely believed, although this has not been established by systematic research, that many dyslexics show distinctive talents in certain areas (compare Geschwind, 1982; West, 1991) and that in general they often show an unusual *balance* of skills. As will be pointed out in the final section of this chapter, this is something which has been partially recognised when diagnostic criteria for dyslexia are specified; but the Harvard research clearly provides a strong taxonomy, and diagnostic criteria that incorporate some of the insights of this research are likely to be more powerful than diagnostic criteria that do not.

(2) Livingstone *et al.* (1991) have distinguished the magnocellular pathways of the visual system from the parvocellular pathways. The former are known in primates to carry fast low-contrast information and the latter slow, high-contrast information. On the basis of experiments involving five dyslexics and the use of visually evoked potentials the authors were led to the suggestion that an important characteristic of dyslexia might be a deficiency in the magnocellular system; and this was confirmed when Galaburda found that in all five of the brains available for *post mortem* examination the magnocellular layers were disorganised and that the cell bodies appeared smaller. Since it is the magnocellular system which is responsible for transmitting information at speed it makes sense to suppose that dyslexics experience difficulty when information has to be processed at high speeds.

(3) Another area of research which is of crucial importance for

the proposed taxonomy is that of genetics (see, for instance, DeFries, 1991; LaBuda and DeFries, 1988). It is now well established that in some – though not all – cases of dyslexia a genetic factor is at work; and where this is so there is an obvious case for lumping.

(4) The work of Livingstone *et al.* (1991) can usefully be linked with that of Tallal (see in particular Tallal, 1980a, b). What Tallal has offered is also, in effect, a proposal for lumping. Some poor readers, on her view, are affected by a mild and subtle form of the kind of language disability which in dysphasics is very much more pronounced. A characteristic which some of her poor readers shared with her dysphasic children was the inability to process auditory stimuli that were presented in quick succession. In one set of experiments the subjects were trained to press one of two panels according to whether the sound presented was high or low in pitch; thereafter they had to press two panels in sequence according to whether pairs of sounds were high–high, low–low, high–low, or low–high. She found that when the two stimuli were separated by 428 ms there were no differences between the poor readers and the controls in the ability to press the correct panel, but that at inter-stimulus-intervals of 8 ms some poor readers, though not all, performed worse than the controls – this despite the fact that the latter were younger. She therefore suggests that in some cases of reading delay there may be difficulty in learning the sounds–symbol relationships that are the basis of phonic rules.

(5) Lovegrove (this volume) distinguishes the transient from the sustained pathways of the visual system, and this appears to be the same distinction as that drawn by Livingstone *et al.* when they speak of the magnocellular and parvocellular pathways. It is not yet known whether there is a similar subdivision in the auditory system; but, as both Lovegrove and Tallal have suggested, if dyslexics since infancy have been at a disadvantage in the processing of speech sounds this would explain how it is that so many of the manifestations of dyslexia can be interpreted as being due to a deficiency in the area of phonology.

(6) No attempt will be made in this chapter to summarise the evidence which supports the idea of such a deficiency. For valuable reviews see Catts (1989) and Rack (this volume). What is important for present purposes is to suggest a further link – that between experiments suggesting a phonological deficiency and the manifestations of dyslexia which have been reported on the basis of

informal observation.

(7) Those who wish for further evidence on these manifestations may like to refer to the many biographical and autobiographical studies in the literature (for references see Miles and Miles, 1990) and to the evidence which has been assembled by Fenwick Stuart (1988) and by Miles (1993a, b). It is noteworthy that for Fawcett, observations of this kind provided the initial stimulus for more systematic research (see Fawcett, preface to this volume). Miles (1988) has spoken of what may be called the 'that's our Johnnie' phenomenon: when the manifestations of dyslexia are suitably described in books or in public lectures parents of dyslexic children regularly notice how the description fits their own child; and this can be seen as an implicit form of lumping, since it is immediately obvious to the parents that the manifestations belong together. There is, on Miles' view, an identifiable *pattern* of difficulties which can easily be picked up after one has carried out a small number of assessments; and he has recently argued (1993a, Chapter 25) that the typical areas of weakness – uncertainty over left and right, difficulty in repeating certain polysyllabic or nonsense words, problems in learning items in series such as the months of the year, and reduced efficiency at recall of auditorily or visually presented digits – can all be understood if one postulates a weakness at what he calls 'verbal labelling' (i.e., a deficit at the phonological level). This weakness can also make sense of dyslexics' slowness at word finding (Spring and Capps, 1974), their lateness in speaking (Done and Miles, 1988), their uncertainties in the area of spoken language (Stirling and Miles, 1988), their difficulty with certain aspects of mathematics (Miles, 1992), and their slowness at reading musical notation (British Dyslexia Association, 1992). What is being suggested here is that no taxonomy of dyslexia can be complete unless the informal observations of parents, teachers and those who carry out assessments are taken into account.

At present the links between these different research areas are suggestive rather than firmly proven. We do not know, for instance, whether those whose dyslexia has been described on the basis of informal observation would, without exception, be found to have symmetrical plana or unusual magnocellular pathways. It would be very exciting if this turned out to be the case.

It should be noted that the proposed taxonomy does not set up 'phonological weakness' in opposition to 'visual weakness'. This is one of the many cases where apparent disagreements can be resolved if we think, not in terms of 'either ... or ...' but rather in terms of 'both ... and ...'. The research of Lovegrove and Tallal straddles this apparent opposition in a particularly interesting way; and, as Stein has pointed out (this volume, p. 149), it is quite possible that 'phonological and visual skills...share a common neurological mechanism'. Whether the phenomena of binocular instability studied by Stein and his colleagues should be lumped with the other dyslexic phenomena or split off from them is a matter that can be resolved only by further research.

Moreover, although the phonological deficit hypothesis plays a major part in the proposed taxonomy it is possible that it will need modification in the future. This will depend, *inter alia,* on the outcome of further work by Nicolson and Fawcett in the area of motor skills (for examples of such work see Chapter 6). If dyslexics turn out to be inferior to controls at motor tasks which demonstrably do not call for any kind of verbal labelling then some wider concept than 'phonological deficit' will be needed. This again, however, is a matter for the future.

There is also the question of whether within the group of dyslexics as at present defined there is any justification for further 'splitting' or subtyping. The supposition that a distinction can be drawn between 'auditory' and 'visual' dyslexics has received a rough ride recently (Liberman, 1985; E. Miles, 1991; Miles and Miles, 1990; Moats, 1991; Ramaa and Lalithamma, 1987); and in the present state of knowledge neither this nor any other form of subtyping has received incontrovertible support. It is not, however, a state of affairs which need be permanent: as was pointed out earlier, advances in knowledge can sometimes lead to further 'splitting', and this is something which may well happen in the case of dyslexia.

There is a possible parallel here with Down's syndrome. Many years after this syndrome was identified it became known that in the great majority of cases those affected had an extra chromosome (47 as opposed to 46). It is now believed that this is true of about 95% of cases (Thomson, 1981). The question arises, therefore, of how to classify the remaining 5%: should they simply be 'lumped' with the other 95% or are they different in respect of a sufficiently large number of characteristics to justify 'splitting' into further separate types? One possibility, it seems, is that Down's syndrome is caused by gene duplication and that individuals with 46 chromosomes carry a duplicated portion of chromosome which produces the same effect as the extra chromosome in 47-chromosome individuals. It is on the basis of this kind of consideration that decisions are made whether to 'lump' or 'split'. Something similar may well be discovered in the case of dyslexia: in particular it is possible that in the future there will have to be 'splitting' between those cases where the dyslexia is hereditary and those where it is not.

The central suggestion in the above proposal for a taxonomy is that there are links between the seven different areas of research which have been mentioned and that no taxonomy can be complete if these links are not recognised. If the taxonomy is along the right lines it may tentatively be claimed that the term 'dyslexia', though it may not have the power of the terms 'tuberculosis' or 'phenylketonuria', nevertheless has more power than the term 'fever' and, *a fortiori*, more power than the term 'excursion-goer'. It also has more power than the term 'poor reading' – a matter which in the present context has important consequences.

CONSEQUENCES FOR TEACHING AND RESEARCH

The consequences for teaching

If those concerned with the teaching of literacy skills choose to concentrate on reading to the exclusion of spelling, essay writing and oral language skills, this could in principle be an informed decision; and in that case no taxonomy other than 'poor reading' would be needed. If, however, the taxonomy of 'poor reading' is adopted in ignorance by educationalists who are unaware of the reasons for the 'dyslexia' taxonomy, they may fail to recognise that spelling, essay writing and oral language skills are also important. Once a person had learned to read there would be no reason in logic to look for other difficulties and their understanding of the position would therefore be incomplete. Nor would they be in a position to increase the dyslexic's understanding of his own difficulties. An inadequate taxonomy can sometimes cause important matters to be overlooked.

The consequences for research

From the point of view of research there is a good case for saying that the concept of 'poor reading' draws the boundaries in the wrong place – that it lumps things that should be kept separate and splits things that should go together. Thus there are poor readers who are not dyslexic (Aaron, 1987; Critchley, 1970; Miles and Haslum, 1986; Stanovich, 1988), and there are many who satisfy some of the other criteria for dyslexia implied by the proposed taxonomy but who nevertheless can read adequately (Miles, 1993a; Miles and Gilroy, 1986; Naidoo, 1972). Moreover the term 'poor reading' diverts attention from the many other difficulties experienced by such individuals – in particular slowness at processing symbolic information (Ellis and Miles, 1977), the persistence of this slowness into adulthood (Miles, 1986), problems of calculation (Miles, 1992), and weakness at getting ideas down on paper (Miles and Gilroy, 1986). The advantage of the dyslexia concept is that it lumps these seemingly disparate manifestations together; and this is precisely what a good taxonomy does. To be a splitter in this area is to miss important links.

The absence of an agreed taxonomy has meant that different investigators have selected their subjects by different criteria; and the position has been made worse by differences in terminology which sometimes – though not always – mask similar selection procedures.

The most common practice is to select children whose reading performance lags behind their age or grade level by more than a specified amount. An intelligence test of some kind is then given so as to ensure that those of low intelligence are excluded from the study, and a check is usually made on other possible adverse factors so that, for example, those with severe personal difficulties and those who are frequently absent from school are also excluded. The remainder then constitute the 'experimental group' and are described either as 'dyslexics' or as 'poor readers'.

This procedure (usually known as 'definition by exclusion') has been criticised on many counts. The basic objection to it is that it lacks adequate taxonomic foundation. The difference between dyslexics and non-dyslexics should in logic be like the difference between those who have phenylketonuria and those who have not, whereas if we are content simply to distinguish poor readers from adequate readers this is like making too much of the distinction between excursion-goers and non-excursion-goers. There need be nothing permanent about a poor reader any more than there is anything permanent about a decision not to go on an excursion. In contrast, if the proposed 'dyslexia' taxonomy is correct, then one would expect at least some of its manifestations to persist over a significant period of time, and even if a particular dyslexic learns to deal adequately with most situations in life one is inclined to say that there has been a learning of 'compensatory strategies' rather than that the dyslexia is no longer present. If the fault lies in the magnocellular pathways of one or more of the sensory systems there may in fact be limits to the extent to which even hard practice can speed up the rate of information processing; and since there is evidence that there are in fact such limits (Miles, 1986) the taxonomy proposal is supported. If one speaks only of 'poor reading' these related findings cannot form part of the picture.

This is not to say that investigations which do not involve strong taxonomies must *ipso facto* be worthless, only that they should not be confused with scientific research. There is nothing wrong with trying to find out if reading standards in one locality are higher or lower than reading standards in another, and the obvious procedure in that case is to obtain reading scores from suitably selected children and make the appropriate statistical comparisons. Such a procedure, however, is not the stuff of which scientific advance is made, and no one should deceive themselves into thinking that it is.

Here are some parallels from other fields. It is clear, for example, that 'oxygen' is a powerful taxonomic term, whereas 'fire', for all its everyday utility, is not. No one is disputing that it would be an entirely justified activity to keep a record of the number of fires that have occurred in a town over the past years; but just because fires occur in accordance with the laws of chemistry such record-keepers cannot claim – and would not wish to claim – that they were doing chemistry as it is currently practised. Similarly, slates fall off roofs if there is a severe storm, and this happens in accordance with the laws of physics; if, however, one collected statistics on the number of slates which fell after a particular storm one could not claim to be doing physics. It is possible that the reason why some pure scientists are sceptical of what they think of as 'social science' research is that they implicitly believe – whether rightly or wrongly – that much of it lacks a proper taxonomic foundation. It would be a pity if this 'blanket' scepticism extended to dyslexia research.

A.W. Ellis (1984) has compared dyslexia with 'stoutness'. If 'dyslexia' is a strong taxonomic term, however, this comparison is inappropriate. Stoutness, as such, clearly does not represent a strong taxonomy, even though a glandular disorder resulting in stoutness would constitute one. If the taxonomy proposed in this chapter is anywhere near correct Ellis's analogy with stoutness is unnecessarily pessimistic, offering, as it does, only a very weak taxonomy.

As is well known, an attempt at an improved classification was made by Rutter and Yule (1975) when they drew a distinction between 'reading backwardness' and 'specific reading retardation'. Whether this classification has any long-term taxonomic power, however, may be doubted. This is because there is nothing in the concept of 'specific reading retardation' to encourage a researcher to look beyond reading performance and apply the kinds of test which the dyslexia concept requires – in particular tests of phonological weakness. Although Rutter and Yule found that those showing 'specific reading retardation' differed in a number of ways from those who were simply 'backward readers' they were unwilling to interpret any of their findings in terms of the dyslexia concept. It is arguable that they were thereby using only a weak taxonomy when a stronger one was in fact available. In scientific research caution is sometimes a virtue, but one may tentatively suggest that in this case it may have inhibited progress!

The difference between the strong taxonomic concept of 'dyslexia' and the relatively weaker concepts of 'backward reading' and 'specific reading retardation' can be further illustrated as follows. (I am grateful to Dr Stanton Newman for calling my attention to this point.) To classify someone as a 'poor reader' involves only a statistical decision about a cut-off point: the result is a stipulation that all those whose scores on one or more reading tests are below this cut-off point shall by definition count as 'poor readers'. In contrast, classifying someone as dyslexic is something which calls for a different methodology. What is needed is that each individual in a survey should be listed separately and that opposite each name there should be columns showing the outcomes of a range of diagnostic tests. The decision 'dyslexic' or 'non-dyslexic' then depends on the overall picture. If one had to rely solely on reading tests it is likely that there would be many more dyslexics on the 'poor reader' side of the cut-off point than on the 'good reader' side; and when research has relied on this criterion the presence of genuine dyslexics may sometimes have produced a significant trend – and therefore valid generalisations about dyslexia – even despite the fact that as a result of inadequate selection procedures a certain amount of unnecessary 'noise' has been introduced into the data. It is, of course, a consequence of the proposed taxonomy that there is no contradiction in saying that a person at the low end of a continuum of reading scores is not dyslexic.

Two further examples may also illustrate how disagreements over the concept of dyslexia are in effect disagreements over the issue of lumping and splitting. It is characteristic of some educational psychologists, presumably because of the wide variety of individual differences that they encounter in their daily practice, to advocate no classification other than 'poor reading'. Thus Whitaker (1989, p. 282) writes: 'The concept is surely..."reading failure" and the examination of this concept must take into account many angles and possible causes'. Similarly Presland (1991, p. 216) writes: 'Is it, indeed, more in keeping with the evidence to distinguish a group of "dyslexics" from other people with reading difficulties or better to think of each person as having an individual pattern of difficulties?'

There is, indeed, no reason to be anything other than a 'splitter' as far as the concept of 'poor reading' is concerned; but it is not clear that Whitaker, Presland, and those who think like them have chosen to be splitters on a secure knowledge base; it seems more likely that they have not fully appreciated the reasons for lumping.

How, then, can selection criteria be specified which are in accordance with the proposed taxonomy?

As was noted above, part of the traditional procedure has been to administer an intelligence test. However, there has been considerable controversy about the reasons for doing so. Particularly significant in this connection are the comments of Stanovich (1991, p. 130) who writes: 'Researchers and practitioners in the field do not seem to have realised that it [sc. intelligence] is a foundation concept for the very idea of dyslexia.' Now it has come to be recognised, chiefly as a result of the writings of Skinner and his followers (see, for example, Skinner, 1953), that all kinds of skills can be learned if one sets about teaching them in the right way; and it follows that to speak of someone's 'not having the intelligence' to do this or that may be unnecessarily defeatist. Indeed, *pace* the writings of Sir Cyril Burt and others (see, for example, Burt, 1955), it is now widely agreed that the concept of intelligence does not have any assured theoretical basis: in the terminology of this chapter, it does not provide a strong taxonomy. Yet if one does not believe in intelligence or IQ in the traditional sense, are there any grounds at all for believing that an intelligence test should play a part in diagnosing dyslexia?

There is the further difficulty that if we examine traditional intelligence tests in detail, we find that they call for a wide variety of different skills. For example, there are items in the Terman Merrill test (Terman and Merrill, 1961) which call both for high-level reasoning and for a knowledge of simple number facts. Thus one of the 'cans of water' items is impossible unless the subject knows, or can work out, that $9 + 4 = 13$, while the 'tree' item is impossible unless the subject knows, or can work out, that $18 + 9 = 27$. Miles (1993a) has reported that among his dyslexic subjects there were some who were capable of the high-level reasoning required by these items but had great difficulty with the number facts. Yet if the objective is an IQ figure based on a strict following of the test instructions, such people – despite their high reasoning power – will have no higher an IQ figure than others for whom the items were simply too difficult. Similarly it is well established that some poor readers and spellers are weak at the four 'ACID' items of the WISC – Arithmetic, Coding, Information and Digit Span (Miles and Ellis, 1981; Naidoo, 1972; Richards, 1985; Rugel, 1974; Spache, 1976), and since Coding is classed as a 'performance' item and the other three as 'verbal' items the value of citing separate figures for 'Verbal IQ', 'Performance IQ', and 'Full Scale IQ' seems highly questionable.

The following would seem to be a possible way forward. What the proposed taxonomy requires is to pick out those individuals in whom the *balance* of skills is unusual. If it can be accepted – perhaps ahead of firm evidence – that the typical dyslexic is weak at what are normally 'left hemisphere' tasks, for instance the ordering and processing of symbols, and strong at right hemisphere tasks such as engineering, computer programming, art and architecture, then such imbalance should be made central to selection procedure. The interesting thing is that this is what discrepancy definitions have largely managed to achieve, albeit at a cost of introducing an appreciable amount of 'noise'. There is 'noise' in that any given research project may have included poor readers who were not dyslexic and will certainly have missed those adequate readers who show other dyslexic signs; and there is further 'noise' in that intelligence may be underestimated if the subject fails a difficult reasoning test only because he does not know, for instance, that 9 + 4 = 13 or performs poorly on the ACID items of the WISC.

There are various ways of reducing this 'noise'. A history of lateness in learning to read is likely to be more informative than a test score administered in a 'one-off' situation; and it may also be useful to take up an idea put forward by Stanovich (1991), viz. that one should measure *listening comprehension* with a view to comparing it with reading skill. In addition, a spelling test may be preferable to a reading test, since although it may generate false positives – those who are poor at spelling but are not dyslexic – it is unlikely to generate any large number of false negatives. This is because learning to spell is harder for dyslexics than learning to read, and it is arguable that anyone who is spelling adequately, if dyslexic at all, at least could not have been all that severely handicapped.

In general it can be said that those who were using discrepancy criteria in picking out dyslexics were doing mostly the right thing, albeit for mostly the wrong reasons. 'Noise' can be reduced if a spelling test is substituted for a reading test, and further evidence for poor phonological skills can be sought if one uses, for example, some of the items in the Bangor Dyslexia Test (Miles, 1982) such as recall of auditorily presented digits, recitation of tables, and repetition of polysyllabic words. In addition, because of possible genetic factors it is very desirable to check on whether anyone else in the family is affected. In adopting these procedures, however, one should not claim to be looking for a discrepancy between reading score and something called 'IQ'; one should rather be using the non-ACID items from the WISC, or tests of reasoning from other intelligence tests, and checking if there is a discrepancy between the subject's reasoning power, as judged by his performance on these items, and his ability to deal with items which are heavy in their phonological demands, such as spelling tests (even more than reading tests) and the items in the Bangor Dyslexia Test.

Any test item if it is to be communicated at all will have at least a minimal phonological component, since the subject needs to be able to identify the symbols which comprise the oral or written instructions, and at least a minimal reasoning component since these instructions have to be understood. Beyond that, however, different items are weighted differently in respect of phonological and reasoning skills. Thus in the Block Design and Object Assembly sub-tests of the WISC a weakness on the phonological side is scarcely a handicap since, understanding the instructions apart, no naming is needed. In 'Similarities' items there is a larger phonological component in that the words have to be identified; but since they are usually words which are within the vocabulary of dyslexics and since there is no time pressure it is entirely appropriate to use Similarities items as tests of reasoning.

The rationale behind the proposed procedure is that the researcher is testing for a possible mismatch between the subjects' reasoning skills on the one hand and their phonological skills on the other. What is being proposed is that those who show this mismatch should be lumped together (and described as 'dyslexic') while in the case of the description 'poor reading' there is no case for being anything other than a splitter.

REFERENCES

Aaron, P.G. (1987). Developmental dyslexia: Is it different from other forms of reading disability? *Annals of Dyslexia, 37*, 109–125.

British Dyslexia Association (1992). *Dyslexia and Music*. Reading: BDA Publications.

Burt, C. (1955). The evidence for the concept of intelligence. *British Journal of Educational Psychology, 25*, 158–177.

Catts, H.W. (1989). Phonological processing deficits and reading disabilities. In A.G. Kamhi and H.W. Catts (Eds.), *Reading Disabilities: A developmental language perspective*. Boston, MA: Little, Brown.

Critchley, M. (1970). *The Dyslexic Child*. London: Heinemann.

Critchley, M. (1978) (Ed.) *Butterworth's Medical Dictionary*. London: Butterworth.

Critchley, M. (1981). Dyslexia: An overview. In G.Th. Pavlidis and T.R. Miles (Eds.), *Dyslexia Research and its Applications to Education*. Chichester: Wiley.

DeFries, J.C. (1991). Genetics and dyslexia: An overview. In M. Snowling and M. Thomson (Eds.), *Dyslexia: Integrating theory and practice*. London: Whurr.

Denckla, M.B. (1972). Clinical syndromes in learning disabilities: The case for 'splitting' vs. 'lumping'. *Journal of Learning Disabilities, 5,* 401–406.

Done, D.J. and Miles, T.R. (1988). Age of word acquisition in developmental dyslexics as determined by response latencies in a picture naming task. In M.M. Gruneberg, L.E. Morris and R.N. Sykes (Eds.), *Practical Aspects of Memory: Current research and issues,* vol. 2, Chichester: Wiley.

Ellis, A.W. (1984). *Reading, Writing, and Dyslexia: A cognitive analysis.* London: Lawrence Erlbaum.

Ellis, N.C. and Miles, T.R. (1977). Dyslexia as a limitation in the ability to process information. *Bulletin of the Orton Society* (now *Annals of Dyslexia*), *27,* 72–81.

Fenwick Stuart, M. (1988). *Personal Insights into the World of Dyslexia.* Cambridge, MA: Educators' Publishing Service Inc.

Galaburda, A.M., Corsiglia, J., Rosen, G.D. and Sherman, G.F. (1987). Planum temporale asymmetry: Reappraisal since Geschwind and Levitsky. *Neuropsychologia, 25,* 853–868.

Galaburda, A.M. Rosen, G.D. and Sherman, G.F. (1989). The neural origin of developmental dyslexia: Implications for medicine, neurology, and cognition. In A.M. Galaburda (Ed.), *From Reading to Neurons.* Cambridge, MA: MIT Press.

Geschwind, N. (1982). Why Orton was right. *Annals of Dyslexia, 32,* 13–30.

Heslop–Harrison, J. (1963). *New Concepts in Flowering and Plant Taxonomy.* London: Heinemann.

Koenigsberg, R. (Ed.) (1989). *Churchill's Medical Dictionary.* New York: Churchill Livingstone.

Labuda, M.C. and DeFries, J.C. (1988). Genetic and environmental etiologies of reading disability: A twin study. *Annals of Dyslexia, 38,* 131–8.

Liberman, I.Y. (1985). Should so-called modality preferences determine the nature of instruction for children with reading disabilities? In F.H. Duffy, and N. Geschwind (Eds.), *Dyslexia: A neuroscientific approach to clinical evaluation.* Boston, MA: Little, Brown.

Livingstone, M., Rosen, G.D., Drislane, F.W. and Galaburda, A.M. (1991). Physiological and anatomical evidence for a magnocellular defect in developmental dyslexia. *Proceedings of the National Academy of Sciences USA, 88,* 7943–7947.

Miles, E. (1991). Visual dyslexia/auditory dyslexia: Is this a valuable distinction to make? In M. Snowling and M. Thomson (Eds.), *Dyslexia: Integrating theory and practice.* London: Whurr.

Miles, T.R. (1982). *The Bangor Dyslexia Test.* Cambridge: Learning Development Aids.

Miles, T.R. (1986). On the persistence of dyslexic difficulties into adulthood. In G.Th. Pavlidis and D.F. Fisher (Eds.), *Dyslexia: Its neuropsychology and treatment.* Chichester: Wiley.

Miles, T.R. (1988). Counselling in dyslexia. *Counselling Psychology Quarterly, 1*, 97–107.

Miles, T.R. (1992). Some theoretical considerations. In T.R. Miles and E. Miles (Eds.), *Dyslexia and Mathematics*. London: Routledge.

Miles, T.R. (1993a). *Dyslexia: The pattern of difficulties*. 2nd edition, London: Whurr.

Miles, T.R. (1993b). *Understanding Dyslexia*. Bath: Amethyst Books.

Miles, T.R. and Ellis, N.C. (1981). A lexical encoding deficiency II. In G.Th. Pavlidis and T.R. Miles (Eds.), *Dyslexia Research and its Applications to Education*. Chichester: Wiley.

Miles, T.R. and Gilroy, D.E. (1986). *Dyslexia at College*. London: Routledge.

Miles, T.R. and Haslum, M.N. (1986). Dyslexia: Anomaly or normal variation? *Annals of Dyslexia, 36*, 103–117.

Miles, T.R. and Miles, E. (1990). *Dyslexia: A hundred years on*. Milton Keynes: Open University Press.

Moats, L.C. (1991). Spelling error interpretation: Beyond the phonetic/dysphonetic dichotomy. *Paper delivered at the Conference of the Orton Dyslexia Society*, Portland, Oregon.

Naidoo, S. (1972). *Specific Dyslexia*. London: Pitman.

Presland, J. (1991). Explaining away dyslexia. *Educational Psychology in Practice, 6*, 215–221.

Ramaa, S. and Lalithamma, M.S. (1987). An alternative explanation to the errors committed by dyslexics while recognising Kannada words. *Paper delivered at the Third World Congress on Dyslexia*, Crete, Greece.

Richards, I.L. (1985). *Dyslexia: A study of developmental and maturational factors associated with a specific cognitive profile*. Unpublished Ph.D. thesis, University of Aston in Birmingham.

Rugel, R.P. (1974). WISC sub–test scores of disabled readers. *Journal of Learning Disabilities, 7*, 48–55.

Rutter, M. and Yule, W. (1975). The concept of specific reading retardation. *Journal of Child Psychology and Psychiatry, 16*, 181–197.

Sherman, G.F., Rosen, G.D. and Galaburda, A.M. (1989). Neuroanatomical findings in developmental dyslexia. In C. Von Euler, I. Lundberg and G. Lennerstrand (Eds.), *Brain and Reading*. Wenner–Gren International Symposium Series, 54.

Skinner, B.F. (1953). *Science and Human Behaviour*. New York: The Free Press; London: Collier–Macmillan.

Spache, G.D. (1976). *Investigating the Issues of Reading Disabilities*. Boston, MA: Allyn and Bacon.

Spring, C. and Capps, C. (1974). Encoding speed, rehearsal, and probed recall of dyslexic boys. *Journal of Educational Psychology, 66*, 780–786.

Stanovich, K.E. (1988). Explaining the differences between the dyslexic and the garden-variety poor reader: The phonological core variable-difference model. *Journal of Learning Disabilities, 21,* 590–612.

Stanovich, K.E. (1991). The theoretical and practical consequences of discrepancy definitions of dyslexia. In M. Snowling and M. Thomson (Eds.), *Dyslexia: Integrating theory and practice.* London: Whurr.

Stirling, E.G. and Miles, T.R. (1988). Naming ability and oral fluency in dyslexic adolescents. *Annals of Dyslexia, 38,* 50–72.

Tallal, P. (1980a). Auditory temporal perception, phonics, and reading disabilities in children. *Brain and Language, 9,* 182–198.

Tallal, P. (1980b). Language and reading: Some perceptual requisites. *Bulletin of the Orton Society* (now *Annals of Dyslexia*), *30,* 170–178.

Terman, L.M. and Merrill, M.A. (1961). *The Revised Stanford Binet Intelligence Scale.* London: H.K. Lewis.

Thomson, W.A.R. (1981). *Black's Medical Dictionary.* London: Black.

Wechsler, D. (1976). *Wechsler Intelligence Scale for Children (WISC–R).* New York: Psychological Corporation.

West, T.G. (1991). *In the Mind's Eye. Visual thinkers, gifted people with learning difficulties, computer images, and the ironies of creativity.* Buffalo, New York: Prometheus Books.

Whitaker, M. (1989). The Bangor Dyslexia Group. *The Psychologist, 2,* 282.

CHAPTER 8

Comparison of deficit severity across skills: Towards a taxonomy for dyslexia

Roderick I. Nicolson and Angela J. Fawcett

INTRODUCTION

In the preceding chapter Miles has argued that an important target for dyslexia research is to develop a 'taxonomy' – a principled classification system based not on arbitrary descriptions of dyslexic performance, but on some underlying causal mechanism. He states that a strong taxonomy implies 'a theory of causation, accurate prognosis, and distinctive methods of treatment' (p. 197). At first sight, the causation criterion appears to correspond with that stated by Rack (Chapter 1). However, in reality the two uses of causality are utterly different. We believe that this is a significant source of theoretical confusion in the literature, responsible for some of the mutual incomprehension between proponents of different viewpoints. When Rack talks about causality, he means 'sufficient to cause the established problems of reading'. This interpretation dates back at least to an influential theoretical analysis by Stanovich (1988), to which we shall return later in this chapter. Most dyslexia researchers have accepted this as a central challenge for theories of dyslexia. Stein and Lovegrove (this volume) implicitly accept this interpretation, and attempt to meet the challenge by demonstrating that visual difficulties may be sufficient to cause the reading problems. By contrast, for Miles the term causality has its traditional scientific usage, namely 'sufficient to cause dyslexia and *all* its symptoms, not just the reading problems'. From Miles' perspective, causality in Stanovich's sense is an interesting but non-central issue. Investigation of the vexed issue of whether or not visual deficits are sufficient in themselves to cause the reading problem may well tell us a great deal about the processes of learning to read. It may not, unfortunately, tell us anything at all about the causes of dyslexia.

Consider now Miles' quotation from Malan on the discovery of the properties of the periodic table (p. 198). This illustrates the standard stages in scientific explanation: namely description, quantification, theory construction, prediction and control. The two initial stages involve data gathering: first developing a clear description of the phenomena involved, and then developing methods for quantifying them, possibly introducing new technical terms and new measurement devices. Failure to undertake this initial exploratory work may result in premature theorising, in which theories are based on incomplete knowledge, and therefore do not cover the full range of phenomena. The next stage involves theory construction, that is, inventing an economical characterisation of the data to be handled in terms of some underlying regularities. For the periodic table, the underlying concepts were in fact mathematical regularities associated with the atomic weights of the elements involved. Once a theory is constructed, it must be tested, first in terms of its sufficiency (to explain the known data), and then, given adequate sufficiency, in terms of its ability to make novel predictions which may then be subjected to empirical tests. Those theories whose predictions are confirmed are then worthy of further development (and the more specific the prediction, or the lower the likelihood of the results being attributable to chance or to other theoretical interpretations, the greater the support for the theory under investigation). It was for this reason that Mendeleyev's predictions, when confirmed, provided such strong support for his theory. Once a theory can make reliable and correct predictions of what will happen under various conditions, the final stage may well be control, that is, ability to manipulate the conditions such that the desired results are obtained. Of course, this bland description of the stages hides the often tortuous and recursive nature of the process. In most areas of scientific endeavour there is usually a period of disconfirmation, when theories' predictions are not supported. This leads to modification and refinement of theories, or in some cases scientific 'revolutions' (Kuhn, 1962), when a completely different perspective is adopted.

As Chomsky (1965) has noted, it is also important to stress the difference between a descriptive theory (such as Mendeleyev's theory of the underlying patterns, or Kepler's theory that the planets travel in ellipsoidal paths around the sun) and a causal, explanatory, theory (for the periodic table, the theory of atomic structure; for the planets, Newton's theory of gravitation). Whilst the development of an adequate descriptive theory is often the appropriate initial target, as Miles notes, true understanding is dependent on developing a causal theory which relates the facts to underlying theoretical knowledge. Until recently it has been rather difficult to determine whether or not a given theory should be deemed explanatory, but in a recent contribution to this rather contentious area of scientific metatheory, Seidenberg (1993, p. 231) argues that one important requirement for an explanatory theory is that it should 'explain phenomena in terms of independently motivated principles'. This distinguishes explanatory theories, such as the atomic weights explanation, from *ad hoc* descriptive theories, such as Mendeleyev's original theory. A further important criterion introduced by Seidenberg (1993, p. 233) is that 'an explanatory theory shows how phenomena previously thought to be unrelated actually derive from a common underlying source.'

From his survey of the dyslexia literature, Miles draws up the range of facts to be considered when attempting to construct a descriptive theory, citing sources of genetic evidence, neuroanatomical evidence, neuropsychological evidence and cognitive evidence (in terms of phonological difficulties and reduced speed of processing). Whilst applauding the general objectives of this approach, which we share, and accepting that Miles' list presents a reasonable overview of the currently available data, we must confess to anxiety about the adequacy of the phenomena cited as the basis for developing even a descriptive theory. If we were to play devil's advocate, we could point out that the various sources of evidence cited by Miles appear unlikely to provide coherent support for any theoretical position. Given the difficulties of linking genes to behaviour, the genetic evidence, for instance, can do little more at present than indicate that the theory must eventually be linked to brain structures, rather than to, say, social circumstances. The neuroanatomical evidence is still preliminary, based on analysis of small numbers of dyslexic and control brains, and, indeed, recent evidence on the issue of symmetry using magnetic resonance imaging (Leonard *et al.*, 1993) suggests that the early research may need reappraisal. Evidence of ectopias and dysplasias appears not to support any specific hypothesis, reflecting instead diffuse microscopic damage throughout the cortex, rather than confined to, say, the language areas (Galaburda, Rosen and Sherman, 1989). There is also evidence of gross cerebral anomalies such as missing or duplicated gyri bilaterally in the planum and parietal operculum (Leonard *et al.*, 1993), though again this appears not to link easily to any specific hypothesis. Evidence for magnocellular deficits in the visual system (Livingstone *et al.*, 1991) is again preliminary, based on small numbers of subjects and, to our knowledge, there is no direct evidence for or against magnocellular deficits in the auditory system, though this is currently an area of intense research activity. Furthermore, there is little available evidence bearing on the critical issue of whether neuroanatomical evidence would distinguish dyslexia from non-specific learning difficulty (low IQ). Turning now to the cognitive deficits, there is clear evidence (as reviewed in this volume) that dyslexic children do show deficits both in processing speed (at least when classification is involved) and in phonological skill. However, it should be emphasised that there is no clear evidence that these deficits distinguish dyslexic children from other groups such as slow learners (low IQ). Indeed, rather the reverse is the case. The bulk of Tallal's research on auditory deficits was in fact undertaken on language-disordered children (e.g., Tallal, Stark and Mellits, 1985). Although language disorder and dyslexia overlap, the majority of dyslexic children would not be classified as language-disordered. More generally, speed of processing deficits correlate highly with low intelligence (Vernon, 1987). There is no doubt that slow learner children suffer from slowness of simple reaction and choice reaction. Perhaps most surprisingly, little attempt appears to have been made to assess the phonological skills of slow learner children. What evidence there is (Shaywitz *et al.*, 1991) suggests that slow learners also have phonological deficits.

It should be stressed that these observations are not intended to belittle the significance of these very important and exciting findings in dyslexia research, they are intended more to sound a note of caution, to raise the possibility that our descriptions are still so incomplete that theorists run a significant risk of premature specificity, and that their theoretical structures will fail to deliver the accurate prognosis demanded of a strong taxonomy. To be even-handed in this devil's advocacy, we note that our own automatisation deficit hypothesis (Chapter 6) is at best a descriptive theory. Furthermore, we have presented no evidence that automatisation deficits do indeed distinguish dyslexic children from slow learners.

In the remainder of this chapter we present an overview of our recently completed research programme, which was designed specifically to remedy these deficits in our knowledge highlighted above by our devil's advocacy.

RESEARCH PROGRAMME

Our research programme started from our work on balance and automatisation and information processing speed (see Chapter 6). In the course of this work, we developed a research design which included six groups of children – three groups of dyslexic children at ages 8, 13 and 17 years, together with three groups of normally achieving children matched for age and IQ. As discussed below, this design allows a number of different analyses to be performed, and provides a method of investigating the effects of maturation on the skills involved. Following these studies, we undertook a range of studies on different primitive skills using the same subject groups as far as possible. Studies included tests of motor skill, tests of phonological skill and tests of naming speed (Fawcett and Nicolson, 1994a, b, c).

We believe that the availability of comprehensive 'across-the-board' data for each participant, together with the availability of between-group statistical analyses, combines the richness of interpretation of case study data with the rigour and generality of traditional experimental designs. The specific issues addressed in the research programme were: first, what proportion of dyslexic children showed each type of deficit; second, whether there is some deficit which is the 'primary' one, which underlies the other deficits; and third, whether it is possible to identify different subtypes of dyslexia, such that each subtype has discriminably different characteristics. Our hope was that the data collected might inform the development of an explanatory framework sufficiently general to accommodate the diversity of the deficits in dyslexia, while sufficiently specific to generate testable predictions, to support better diagnostic procedures, and to inform remediation methods.

Participants

There is considerable controversy over methods of defining dyslexia, and in particular whether it is appropriate to differentiate between dyslexic children and *slow learners* – poor readers whose reading is nonetheless at about the level of the rest of their attainments (Siegel, 1989; Stanovich, 1991). This issue is by no means resolved, but, regardless of the final outcome, the only way to establish evidence relevant to the distinction is to maintain it. Consequently, since we wished to study *pure dyslexia*, in selecting our dyslexic groups we used the standard exclusionary criterion of 'children of normal or above normal intelligence – operationalised as IQ of 90 or more on the WISC-R (Wechsler, 1976) – without known primary emotional or behavioural or socioeconomic problems, and whose reading age (RA) was at least 18 months behind their chronological age (CA)'. We recruited three groups of dyslexic children, with mean ages 17, 13 and 8 years, together with three groups of normal children matched for age and IQ. This gave us six groups, D17, D13 and D8; and C17, C13 and C8 for the three age groups of dyslexic and control children respectively. The dyslexic children were located via the local Dyslexia Institute or the local branch of the British Dyslexia Association. Other than checking that the children met our criteria for dyslexia, and that they were willing to undertake testing on a long-term basis, no screening or selection whatsoever was undertaken. This three-age-group design allows performance to be compared with children of the same age (D17 vs C17; D13 vs C13; D8 vs C8), children of around the same reading age (D17 vs C13; D13 vs C8) and children of around half the age (D17 vs C8). The issue of whether dyslexia is discriminably different from slow learning was partially addressed by recruiting a seventh group of slow learners (SL10), of age 10 years, matched for reading ability with the D8 group, but with IQ (WISC-R) in the range 70–90.

Skill tests

One of the problems of investigating a disorder of reading is that the process of reading is so complex, requiring the fluent interplay of a number of subskills together with the smooth integration of lexical, phonological and orthographic knowledge. A deficit in any or all of these components would lead to problems in learning to read. Furthermore, since reading is a crucial school attainment, considerable and varied efforts may be made to train the component skills, and this differential training experience leads to further difficulties in interpretation of any differences in reading ability. In an attempt to minimise confounding factors arising from differences in experience together with use of compensatory strategies, we decided to test primitive skills in the major modalities – skills which are not normally trained explicitly, and are not easily subject to compensatory strategies. In order to standardise testing techniques and to facilitate replication by other researchers, these tests were implemented where possible on an Apple Macintosh computer, using digitised sound for instructions and stimuli, and using automatic event recording and data analysis techniques. In addition to psychometric tests, five generic types of test were used, namely tests of phonological skill, working memory, information processing speed, motor skill and sensory estimation. The psychometric tests used the WISC-R scales (Wechsler, 1976), with spelling age and reading age based on the Schonell tests of single word reading and spelling. The tests of phonological skill included phonological discrimination ability for phonologically confusable stimuli (Bishop, 1985), segmentation ability (Rosner and Simon, 1971) and 'rhyming' ability for phonemes at the beginning, middle and end of words (a simplified version of the tests used in Bradley and Bryant, 1983). The working memory tests included nonword repetition (repeating nonsense words of 2, 3, 4 and 5 syllables – based on Gathercole and Baddeley, 1990), the mean Memory Span for words of 1, 2 and 3 syllables, and articulation rate (the mean of the times to repeat five times *bus, monkey* and *butterfly,* respectively), which is included in this category because memory span and articulation rate are known to co-vary (Baddeley, Thomson and Buchanan, 1975). Tests of information processing speed included: tests of speed of naming of pictures, colours, digits and letters (all presented unpaced); simple reaction and selective choice reaction time to pure tones; visual search (locating a distinctive spotty dog on each of several crowded pages in a child's puzzle book), and tachistoscopic word recognition on a graded series of words presented for gradually decreasing times ('Word Flash'). The motor skill tests included tests of bead threading and pegboard peg moving together with a variety of static balance tasks. These included standing on both feet, standing on one foot, standing on both feet when blindfolded, standing on one foot while blindfolded, and dual task balance, which involved standing on one (or two) feet while undertaking a secondary, choice reaction, task. The dependent variable for the balance tasks was the number of wobbles occurring within one minute (30 s for one foot balance). A final set of tests was developed in order to investigate sensory estimation ability. Three tests were used: temporal estimation, in which two tones were presented one second apart, and the subject had to specify which one was of longer duration; line estimation, in which two lines were presented, one second apart, and the subject had to specify which one was the longer; and loudness estimation, in which two tones were presented, one second apart, and the subject had to specify which one was the louder. The tests were based directly on those presented in Ivry and Keele (1989). The variable of interest in the three tests was the 'threshold' at which subjects could just detect the difference. The computer-based versions of all the tests are available in the COMB set (Nicolson, 1993).

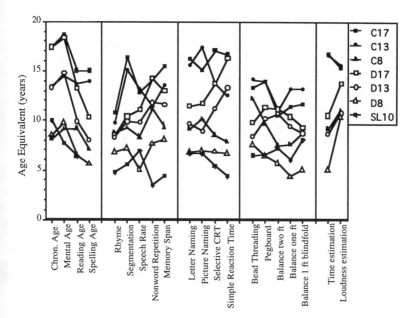

Figure 8.1 Comparative performance of the seven groups on selected tests

RESULTS

Detailed presentations of results and procedures for the different types of skill are given in Fawcett and Nicolson (1994a, b, c); Nicolson, Fawcett and Dean (1994). In order to facilitate visual comparison between tests, the results for each test have been converted to the age-equivalent scores, taking the data from our control groups together with control data from other studies where possible (Figure 8.1). Looking just at the three control groups (filled symbols), performance on the psychometric tests improves with age, as expected. With age there is also better phonological discrimination and segmentation; roughly equivalent rhyming performance; better performance on memory span, and especially articulation rate; faster processing; and better performance on the single task balance. Performance is roughly equivalent on fine motor skill (beads and pegs). Whenever there is a difference, the oldest controls performed the best, and the youngest controls the worst. In other words, the results for control groups are largely as one would expect, with some of the skills still developing in the teens, and some (such as the beads test and the rhyming test) already at ceiling (at least on the tests used).

Now consider the performance of the dyslexic groups (open symbols). The psychometric data are largely as expected, since the pairs of groups were matched for IQ and age. As expected, reading age lagged further and further behind chronological age, with an even greater deficit for spelling age. Phonological skills indicate marked deficits, with the D8 group showing the expected lag, and surprisingly poor performance for the D17 group, comparable to that of the C8 group. In segmentation and rhyming the dyslexic children performed significantly worse than their reading age controls. Note also the severe deficits of the D8 group in the memory and articulation skills, but in this case the three dyslexic groups show a heartening developmental trend, with the abysmal performance of the D8 group making way to merely poor performance of the D13s and near-adequate performance of the D17s. A similar pattern of performance is shown for the tests of processing speed (with the exception of the simple reactions, where the dyslexic children performed at normal standards). In contrast to the other tests, the D17s consistently outscored the C8s on these tests of memory and processing speed. Most notable overall is the extraordinarily poor performance of all three dyslexic groups on the motor skill tasks, in particular one foot balance and blindfold balance. Indeed, the D8 group were performing at only the 4-year-old level on the balance tasks, and since our norms only go down to 3.5 years this is very poor performance indeed.

In almost all tests of naming speed, phonological skill, motor skill, and also nonword repetition and articulation rate, the dyslexic children performed significantly worse than their chronological age controls. In general, the performance of the dyslexic children was somewhat below that of their reading age controls, but significant differences compared with reading age controls were obtained only for simple reaction (better performance than the reading age controls) and phonological skills, picture naming speed, bead threading and balance under dual task conditions or when blindfolded (worse than reading age controls). Furthermore, it may also be seen that the performance of the oldest dyslexic children is by no means better overall than that of the youngest controls, despite the advantage of around nine years' experience.

Comparison with slow learners

The comparisons between the D8 group and the SL10 group are also very interesting. The slow learners performed significantly the better only for balance, whereas they were significantly worse on phonological skills, memory span and simple reaction time. Performance on the other tasks was comparable for both groups. There appears to be an interesting anomaly on articulation rate (see Figure 8.1) in that there is a dissociation from the other phonological and memory tasks, in which the slow learners performed significantly worse, whereas for articulation rate they performed noticeably (but not significantly) better.

Individual differences in dyslexia

One of the major issues in dyslexia research is the degree of specificity of the different facets of deficit. Boder (1973) argued for a distinction between visual and phonological subtypes of dyslexia, a distinction that has led to enduring controversy in the literature, with a schism between the 'lumpers' (who argue that there is a single underlying cause, although it may be manifested in different ways) and the 'splitters' (who argue that it is better to treat dyslexia as a collection of subtypes). This type of debate has proved unproductive in other domains (such as intelligence), but there is a significant applied issue. If, for instance, there is an important distinction to be made between visual and phonological dyslexia, it seems likely that different remediation approaches should be adopted for each subtype. If, on the other hand, there is a single set of causes, it is likely that generic remediation methods may be developed. See Miles (this volume) for further thoughts on this theme.

In an initial attempt to address this issue we conducted principal components analyses on the data. Unfortunately, the ratio of subjects to variables is only around 2.5, below the recommended

Dyslexia in Children

minimum of 3 (Barrett and Kline, 1981). Not surprisingly, therefore, the factor structure was unstable, with small changes in analysis method and/or tests included leading to radically different structures, many involving implausible collections of seemingly disparate tests.

Consequently, we performed an analysis of the pattern of individual performance across the types of skill tested. This was undertaken by first normalising the data for each test for each group relative to that of the corresponding control group. For example, for the D17 group the data for blindfold balance for each subject were normalised by obtaining the difference of the datum from the mean blindfold balance score for group C17, and then dividing this difference by the standard deviation of the C17 group for blindfold balance. Groups D17 and C17 were normalised relative to C17, groups D13 and C13 were normalised relative to C13, and groups C8, D8 and SL10 were normalised relative to C8. This procedure led to what was essentially an age-appropriate 'effect size' in standard deviation units (analogous to a z-score) for each test for each child. A child was deemed to be 'at risk' on a given task if his or her effect size on that task was −1 or worse. The median effect sizes (averaged across age levels) and incidence (the proportion of at risk children), ranked in order of decreasing effect size severity for the dyslexic groups, are collated in Table 8.1. [1]

Inspection of Table 8.1 indicates that most of the dyslexic children were impaired on a wide range of tasks. Naturally they were all impaired on reading since this was a requirement for inclusion in the dyslexia groups; and the even greater impairment in spelling than reading is as expected (Thomson, 1984). The other tasks for which the median effect size was −2 or worse are balance (dual task, one foot blindfold, and one foot non-blindfold), segmentation, letter naming speed, time estimation and articulation rate, with an incidence rate of around 80% on most of these skills. Indeed, of the 30 dyslexic children who completed at least three of the five tasks (dual task balance, one foot blindfold balance, segmentation, letter naming and time estimation) 24 (80%) had positive scores on at least three. Of the remaining 6 children, 3 showed deficits on two of the tasks. By contrast, only 1 out of the 37 controls completing at least three of the tasks showed a deficit on three or more tasks, and a further 2 showed two deficits.

Table 8.1 Incidence of dyslexia 'at risk' scores in the three groups
(in decreasing order of effect size severity)

Task	Dyslexic		Control		Slow Learner	
	Effect size.	Incid-ence	Effect size	Incid-ence	Effect size	Incid-ence
Spelling Age	−5.60	35/36	−0.17	5/39	—	—
Balance Dual	−5.38	21/25	0.23	5/32	—	—
Reading Age	−3.72	36/36	−0.38	5/39	−2.54	11/11
Balance 1 foot blindfold	−3.31	27/33	−0.06	4/31	−0.14	3/11
Segmentation	−3.11	21/25	0.26	2/32	−5.76	10/11
Letter Naming Speed	−2.66	22/28	0.11	4/33	−2.82	10/11
Time Estimation	−2.38	24/30	0.12	6/36	−7.02	—
Articulation Rate	−2.32	20/36	0.10	6/31	−0.61	4/11
Balance 1 foot	−2.11	23/33	0.22	7/31	−1.23	7/11
Balance 2 foot blindfold	−1.84	15/34	0.43	5/31	−0.56	1/11
Picture Naming Speed	−1.65	20/28	−0.06	5/33	−2.51	9/11
Digit Naming Speed	−1.53	20/28	0.25	5/33	−1.96	10/11
Lexical Decision Time	−1.49	13/36	0.18	6/36	−0.85	3/11
Word Flash	−1.43	18/27	0.01	6/32	—	—
Line Estimation	−1.30	18/30	0.16	4/36	−0.44	—
Colour Naming Speed	−1.26	14/28	0.30	4/33	−0.94	3/11
Pegs	−1.23	11/29	0.13	5/31	−1.97	10/11
Selective Choice RT	−1.18	18/36	−0.06	5/33	−0.73	5/11
Beads	−1.12	8/29	0.16	4/29	−1.63	8/11
Rhyme	−0.96	17/27	0.17	4/33	−3.70	11/11
Visual Search	−0.87	12/24	0.10	4/33	—	—
Phon. Discrimination	−0.63	14/36	0.23	6/31	—	—
Memory Span	−0.45	11/36	−0.01	5/31	−2.25	11/11
Loudness Estimation	−0.43	7/27	0.22	6/35	—	—
Nonword Repetition	−0.39	12/36	0.24	4/31	−12.61	11/11
Balance Both Feet	0.02	7/34	0.37	5/31	0.19	1/11
Simple RT	0.07	10/36	0.23	6/33	−1.86	7/11

It seems clear, therefore, that in the dyslexic children that we investigated, the considerable majority showed deficits in many of the primitive skills tested. If there are pure phonological dyslexics, they are poorly represented in our sample. Inspection of the individual data revealed that, of the 33 dyslexic children who attempted both one foot blindfold balance and dual task balance, only 3 (2 in the D15 group, and 1 in the D8 group) were not scored at risk on either task. Even these 3 showed a deficit in two feet blindfold balance. Balance difficulties, especially when blindfolded, appear therefore to be associated with all our sample of dyslexic children.

Turning now to a comparison with the slow learners, Table 8.1

indicates an interesting dissociation. Both the dyslexic and slow learner groups performed very poorly on the phonological tasks and the naming tasks. Interestingly, the slow learners performed exceptionally poorly (significantly worse than the dyslexic children) on the phonological tasks, with an effect size on nonword repetition of −12.6. The slow learners also performed poorly on the dexterity tasks (beads and pegs), the memory span and the simple reaction task. By contrast, the slow learners showed little deficit on the balance tasks and on the articulation time.

DISCUSSION

Before attempting a theoretical interpretation of these results, it is important to attempt to characterise them, in order to provide a set of requirements for theorists wishing to develop their own accounts of the data.

Breadth of deficit

Deficits were observed in *all* the primitive skills tested – phonological, speed, memory and motor skill. There is no support here for any of the theories that attempt to tie dyslexia to one specific modality or type of process. The statistical comparisons showed that, in general, the dyslexic children were performing at or around the level of their reading age controls for speed of information processing and for memory, and below reading age for motor skill and phonological skill.

Changes with age

The most striking aspect of our data is the range of very profound deficits suffered by the youngest dyslexic children. Figure 8.1 does not really capture these particularly well, because many of the youngest dyslexic children had a performance well below the 4-year-old age norm, especially for phonological skill and motor skill.

Following this very poor start, the dyslexic children actually make pretty good progress in speed of processing and in memory, possibly even catching up a bit. By contrast, there remain deficits in phonological skill and especially in balance, as shown by the performance of the D17 group. This pattern of results suggests that the learning processes are essentially intact, but that skill acquisition is greatly hampered by the initial very poor performance. This interpretation is strengthened by the results of experiments in which we investigated acquisition of skill directly, by undertaking a long-term training study in which we studied the blending of two simple reactions (a finger press to a tone and a foot press to a flash) into a choice reaction (see Study 4, Chapter 6, this volume). Here we found that although each individual simple reaction was at normal speed, the dyslexic group were very much slower than the controls when the two simple reactions were first combined as a choice reaction. They then showed reasonably normal improvement in the skill with practice, but even so, at the end of 25 sessions' practice (some 5,000 trials) the dyslexic group were significantly slower than the controls, and more error-prone. Furthermore, whereas the controls had reached their baseline simple reaction speed following this extended practice on choice reactions, the dyslexic group still fell significantly short of the baseline speed.

Specific difficulties

Although it is clear that there are problems in all primitive skills, it is also important to identify which types of skill show the greatest deficits, since this may give some clue as to the most likely cause(s). As noted above, phonological skill and motor skill appear to be least susceptible to improvement with age (with significant deficits even compared with reading age controls on several phonological and motor tasks), with information processing speed and memory showing the greatest improvement. It is also important to consider, within each modality, which type of skill is most affected. Consider first speed of reaction. Here we found that simple reactions were essentially normal, but that problems arose as soon as a decision was required (selective choice reaction). Irrespective of the reason for the apparently normal speed of simple reaction, the choice reaction deficit occurred whether or not linguistic stimuli were involved, and regardless of whether the stimuli were visual or auditory. Now consider motor skill. There were severe initial deficits in bead threading, pegboard manipulation and normal balance, but the latter two did at least improve with age. By contrast, the deficit in blindfold balance persisted into the D17 group, with performance worse than that of the C8 group. In phonological skill it is clear that the deficit in segmentation remained into adolescence.

INTERPRETATION

Before turning to our interpretation of the results, it is important to address a theoretical paradox highlighted in an influential analysis by Stanovich (1988). The 'assumption of specificity'– that 'the cognitive problems characteristic of the dyslexic child are reasonably specific to the reading task and do not implicate broader domains of cognitive functioning' (p. 154) – is a central tenet of many dyslexia researchers. However, cognitive research had uncovered a range of deficits on cognitive tasks including metacognitive functioning. Stanovich asserts:

> Further developments along these lines will surely develop into a paradoxical conclusion: that reading-disabled [dyslexic] children are deficient in a generalized ability to deal with cognitive tasks of all types (i.e., they lack metacognitive awareness: a critical aspect of intelligence). This, of course, would be the death knell for the assumption of specificity, and hence the entire rationale for the concept of reading disability would be undermined. (p. 157)

Stanovich attempts to retain the assumption of specificity by questioning the cognitive deficit findings, and suggests such findings may be artifactual, either because the deficits may derive from lack of motivation and/or opportunity arising from reading failure (the Matthew effect), or because the results may derive from inclusion of slow learners within the dyslexic sample, or because there is in reality a continuum between dyslexia and slow learning. He asserts that the best candidates for key processing mechanisms underlying reading disability will be non-central, modular mechanisms, and he develops the argument that one key to fluent reading is the development of an autonomously functioning module at the word recognition level, and that failure to develop such a module may derive from impairments in phonological processing.

Forewarned by Stanovich's analysis, we designed the research programme so as to provide a sharp examination of the assumption of specificity. Our selection procedures explicitly distinguished between slow learners and dyslexic children. By investigating primitive skills, on which it is hard to improve or impair performance by means of cognitive set or strategy adoption, and for which there was typically no right answer, we hoped to limit the possible effects of negative expectations. By investigating a range of skills, some related to reading and/or schoolwork and some not, we hoped to control for the possibility of differential practice and/or differential motivation. Finally, by investigating developmental changes in performance we intended to assess the cumulative nature of the deficit. If the Matthew effect is the sole cause of deficits in areas not directly related to reading, one would expect an increase of impairment with age, owing to the cumulative vicious circle involved.

The results of our research programme cause grave difficulties for the assumption of specificity. Dissociations between performance of the slow learners and the dyslexic children were obtained on several tasks. Deficits compared with same age controls were found across the range of primitive skills, with the sole exception of simple reactions. Individual analyses suggested a surprising homogeneity in the deficits, with almost all the dyslexic children exhibiting the key symptoms. It is hard to believe that the Matthew effect could impair balance or time estimation performance whilst leaving simple reactions unimpaired. Finally, deficits typically decreased with age. The results therefore do completely undermine the assumption of specificity.[2] We do not accept, however, that they undermine the 'entire rationale for the concept of reading disability'. The challenge, which we shall meet below, is to develop a framework which accounts for the range of deficits shown by dyslexic children but which does not involve a central cognitive impairment.

First, though, let us return to the initial motivations for our research programme: to establish what proportion of dyslexic children showed deficits in the various primitive skills tested; to assess the evidence for subtypes of dyslexia; and to investigate which if any of the deficits is the primary one. On the first two issues the results are remarkably clear-cut. The dyslexic children showed deficits across the spectrum of primitive skills, and there was no evidence for subtypes of dyslexia, at least within the sample investigated. In terms of the primary deficit, the answer will depend upon both the level of explanation sought and the purpose of the enquiry. It may well be, for instance, that in terms of acquisition of reading skill, the primary deficit is indeed that of phonological skill (Bradley and Bryant, 1983). It also appears that if one had to characterise the qualitative aspects of performance, a parsimonious description is given in terms of an automatisation deficit (Nicolson and Fawcett, 1990), in that the deficits across the spectrum of primitive skill are precisely as predicted by the automatisation deficit hypothesis.

Interestingly, the automatisation deficit account also fulfils Stanovich's dual criteria for a causal theory of dyslexia. It explains naturally why dyslexic children are impaired in the 'development of an autonomously functioning module at the word recognition level'. Furthermore, it allows that central cognitive processes, such as metacognition, are completely unimpaired, thereby explaining the average or above average intelligence. Nonetheless, the hypothesis is the precise opposite of the assumption of specificity, suggesting instead an *assumption of generality,* where performance deficits are expected on any skill which requires automatisation. Apparently normal performance is accounted for in terms of conscious compensation, or at least more effortful processing. We suggest that the logical flaw in Stanovich's argument is the implicit assumption that there can be only one form of 'central' factor underlying reading deficits, namely a high-level cognitive factor. Learning is an alternative central factor, and although it is likely that a deficit in symbolic learning would lead to reduced intelligence, any deficit in low-level, sub-symbolic learning could lead to precisely the range of symptoms obtained. Indeed, in Nicolson and Fawcett (1994b) we proposed that the deficits shown in our long-term training studies were best modelled not as difficulties in automatisation *per se*, but rather as consistent with greater neural noise, which causes difficulties in sub-symbolic learning, leading to marked initial deficits, normal rate of acquisition of skill, but slower, more effortful and more error-prone performance on any primitive skill. It should also be noted that the automatisation deficit hypothesis satisfies Seidenberg's two criteria for explanatory theories (see

Introduction), namely explanation in terms of independently motivated theories, and showing how phenomena previously thought to be unrelated derive from a common underlying source.

However, despite these striking successes, neither the automatisation deficit hypothesis nor the neural noise hypothesis truly attacks the underlying cause, and we feel that both accounts are probably better seen as descriptive theories – attempts to describe the symptoms of dyslexia economically from the perspectives of cognitive psychology and connectionist learning respectively. A causal explanation should account for the precise pattern of results obtained, and should identify the mechanism(s) underlying these symptoms. At this stage that we relax scientific caution, and put forward a speculation which is by no means fully established as yet. The speculation centres on new findings concerning the role of the cerebellum in cognition. We are indebted to our colleague Paul Dean for alerting us to this literature, and for collaborating with us on the research reported in the following section.

Speculation on the role of the cerebellum in dyslexia

Phonological skill, blindfold balance and time estimation skills not only show a marked deficit at age 8 years, but also appear resistant to maturational improvement, to the extent that the oldest dyslexic children have barely reached the performance level of the youngest controls. Clearly, if there were some mechanism underlying the deficits in balance, time estimation and phonological skill, that mechanism would be a prime candidate for the underlying cause of dyslexia.

The deficit in balance (especially blindfold balance) suggests some disorder of the vestibular system or the cerebellum. The cerebellum is also implicated by its supposed involvement in the automatisation of motor skill and procedural learning (Ito, 1984; 1990). Levinson (1990), on the basis of studies of nystagmus and optokinetic fixation in dyslexic children, has for some time argued for mild cerebellar dysfunction as a causal factor in dyslexia. However, the traditional view of cerebellar function (Eccles, Ito and Sventagothai, 1967) is as a centre for motor skill rather than cognitive skill, and so the cerebellum has been discounted as a potential causal factor by most dyslexia researchers. Recently, however, there has been a series of studies and reviews (Leiner, Leiner and Dow, 1989; 1993) which suggest strongly that the human cerebellum is in fact closely involved in cognitive skill as well as motor skill. The authors put forward the 'Cognitive Cerebellum' hypothesis, that the neocerebellum is centrally involved in cognitive skill acquisition:

> The mammalian cerebellum seems able to improve the skilled performance of any cerebral area to which it is linked by 2-way neural connections ... the 2-way connections linking the cerebellum to Broca's area make it possible for the cerebellum to improve language dexterity, which combines motor and mental skills. (1989, p. 1007)

This claim is not yet fully established (Glickstein, 1993; for a recent debate see Leiner, Leiner and Dow, 1993). Nonetheless, the hypothesis provides a natural explanation of the deficits in 'language dexterity' which underlie the known phonological deficits. It was, in fact, for this reason that we undertook the stimulus comparison studies of time estimation, line estimation and loudness estimation. The design was based on studies by Ivry and Keele (1989), who demonstrated that patients with cerebellar lesions were specifically impaired on time estimation but not loudness estimation, whereas neither Parkinson's nor patients with cortical neuropathy showed a deficit in time estimation. The cerebellar deficit hypothesis predicted a dissociation between temporal estimation and loudness estimation, whereas, to our knowledge, no other theory of dyslexia made such a prediction. It should be noted, for instance, that the theory of impaired rapid processing would predict no impairment, since the temporal judgement is certainly not mediated by the magnocellular pathways. The predicted dissociation was obtained, with the dyslexic groups showing significant impairment (even compared with reading age controls) on temporal estimation, whereas the deficits on loudness estimation were small and non-significant. These findings are confirmed by the effect size of −2.38 and incidence of 80% for temporal estimation, contrasted with the effect size of only −0.43 and incidence of 26% for loudness estimation (Table 8.1). Confirmation of the predictions, together with the magnitude of the effect size for temporal estimation, among the largest in our research programme, therefore provide strong support for the role of the cerebellum in dyslexia (Nicolson, Fawcett and Dean, 1994).

It may be seen, therefore, that the hypothesis of dysfunction in the cerebellum or its neural tracts provides a natural explanation of the three major deficits (balance, phonological skill and temporal estimation) obtained in this series of studies. Furthermore, such a hypothesis accounts naturally for our finding (Nicolson and Fawcett, 1994b) that dyslexic children have problems *initially* in blending two skills but that subsequent skill acquisition is not abnormal save for difficulties in error elimination, in that a PET study (Roland *et al.*, 1989) has identified activation of the cerebellum in learning but not recognition; a case study of cerebellar damage has revealed specific difficulties in cognitive learning and error detection (Fiez *et al.*, 1992), and a cerebellar inactivation study in rabbits (Krupa, Thompson, and Thompson, 1993) has indicated that the cerebellum is particularly involved in initial skill acquisition.

Even so, the link with the cerebellum is speculative at this stage, and further research is needed to test the hypothesis. The neuroanatomical findings of deficits in the magnocellular pathways, together with diffuse cortical abnormalities identified by Galaburda and his colleagues, suggest that it will not be the only abnormal brain structure. We put forward the hypothesis as an illustration of the new research avenues suggested by the findings presented here, and as a demonstration that it is possible to abandon Stanovich's assumption of specificity without undermining the concept of dyslexia.

CONCLUSIONS

In conclusion, we believe that the studies in this chapter present the most complete picture to date of skills in dyslexic children. The results provide very strong evidence that dyslexic children suffer from problems in a range of primitive skills, and that the underlying cause(s) must lie deep within central brain function.

We believe that the concept of automatisation deficit provides the basis for a valuable descriptive theory of the causes of dyslexia, lacking only the link to underlying neural structures to be a true, explanatory theory. To return briefly to three requirements of a strong taxonomy stated by Miles, we have a theory of causation; this in turn promises development of more accurate methods of prognosis (diagnosis), suggesting methods not only for distinguishing dyslexic children from non-dyslexic children and from slow learners, but also suggesting methods for diagnosis of dyslexia before children try (and fail) to learn to read. The theory does suggest distinctive methods of remediation (in terms of greater systematicity in teaching the necessary subskills before complex skills are taught), but these methods reflect existing good practice in the area (E. Miles, 1989).

We have presented strong preliminary evidence that the cerebellum might be the brain structure mediating the difficulties in automatisation and in phonological skill. This hypothesis satisfies Miles' requirements for a strong dichotomy, it satisfies Seidenberg's requirements for an explanatory theory, it satisfies Stanovich's requirements for a causal explanation of dyslexia, it provides an excellent general account of both the qualitative pattern and the quantitative detail of the results obtained in the study reported here, and it has already proved fruitful, generating a novel and unique prediction which was confirmed by a stringent empirical test.

We have only just begun to explore the cerebellar deficit hypothesis. It may be wrong in detail or in principle. Nonetheless, right or wrong, we believe that it illustrates better than any hypothetical example the potential benefits to dyslexia research of having a strong taxonomy. We hope and expect that other researchers will shortly propose alternative theories for the data we have presented here, and the data which have been reported throughout this book. This is the essence of scientific progress.

ACKNOWLEDGEMENTS

The research reported here was supported by grants from the Leverhulme Trust and the Medical Research Council to the University of Sheffield. We thank Paul Dean for alerting us to the possible role of the cerebellum in dyslexia, and for comments on an early draft. We also wish to thank Alan Baddeley and Tim Miles for valuable suggestions for the design of the studies. We acknowledge gratefully the dedicated support of the participants and their parents.

Notes

[1]   The precise values of the effect sizes depend critically upon the standard deviation of the corresponding control group for the task in question. In view of the small number of subjects in each group, together with the relative homogeneity of the control groups, the effect size data should be interpreted with caution. Nonetheless, the effect size analysis provides a valuable method of comparing across tasks for the same subject population.

[2]   We do not suggest, however, that the Matthew effect is not important. Anyone who has seen the corrosive effects of reading failure on self-esteem and school performance of a child with dyslexia will appreciate the power of Stanovich's analysis. The issue is whether the Matthew effect alone is sufficient to account for the non-reading difficulties suffered by children with dyslexia. Our results indicate that they are not.

REFERENCES

Baddeley, A.D., Thomson, N. and Buchanan, M. (1975). Word length and the structure of short-term memory. *Journal of Verbal Learning and Verbal Behavior, 14,* 575–589.

Barrett, P. and Kline, P. (1981). The observation to variable ratio in factor analyses. *Journal of Personality and Group Psychology, 1,* 23–33.

Bishop, D. (1985). Spelling ability in congenital dysarthria: Evidence against articulatory coding in translating between graphemes and phonemes. *Cognitive Neuropsychology, 2,* 229–251.

Boder, E. (1973). Developmental dyslexia: A diagnostic approach based on three atypical spelling–reading patterns. *Developmental Medicine and Child Neurology, 15,* 663–687.

Bradley, L. and Bryant, P.E. (1983). Categorising sounds and learning to read: A causal connection. *Nature, 301,* 419–421.

Chomsky, N. (1965). *Aspects of the Theory of Syntax.* Dordrecht, Netherlands: Foris.

Eccles, J.C., Ito, M. and Szentagothai, J. (1967). *The Cerebellum as a Neuronal Machine.* New York: Springer-Verlag.

Fawcett, A.J. and Nicolson, R.I. (1994a). Persistent deficits in motor skill for children with dyslexia. *Journal of Motor Behavior.* In press.

Fawcett, A.J. and Nicolson, R.I. (1994b). Persistent deficits in phonological skill for older dyslexic children. Submitted.

Fawcett, A.J. and Nicolson, R.I. (1994c). Naming speed in children with dyslexia. *Journal of Learning Disabilities.* In press.

Fiez, J.A., Petersen, S.E., Cheney, M.K. and Raichle, M.E. (1992). Impaired non-motor learning and error detection associated with cerebellar damage: A single case study. *Brain, 112,* 155–178.

Galaburda, A.M., Rosen, G.D. and Sherman, G.F. (1989). The neural origin of developmental dyslexia: Implications for medicine, neurology and cognition. In A.M. Galaburda (Ed.), *From Reading to Neurons* (pp. 377–388). Cambridge, MA: MIT Press.

Gathercole, S.E. and Baddeley, A.D. (1990). Phonological memory deficits in language disordered children: Is there a causal connection? *Journal of Memory and Language, 29,* 336–360.

Glickstein, M. (1993). Motor skills but not cognitive tasks. *Trends in Neuroscience, 16,* 450–451.

Ito, M. (1984). *The Cerebellum and Motor Control.* New York: Raven Press.

Ito, M. (1990). A new physiological concept on cerebellum. *Revue Neurologique (Paris), 146,* 564–569.

Ivry, R.B. and Keele, S.W. (1989). Timing functions of the cerebellum. *Journal of Cognitive Neuroscience, 1,* 136–152.

Krupa, D.J., Thompson, J.K. and Thompson, R.F. (1993). Localization of a memory trace in the mammalian brain. *Science, 260,* 989–991.

Kuhn T. (1962). *The Structure of Scientific Revolutions.* Chicago: University of Chicago Press.

Leiner, H.C., Leiner, A.L. and Dow, R.S. (1989). Reappraising the cerebellum: What does the hindbrain contribute to the forebrain? *Behavioural Neuroscience, 103,* 998–1008.

Leiner, H.C., Leiner, A.L. and Dow, R.S. (1993). Cognitive and language functions of the human cerebellum. *Trends in Neuroscience, 16,* 444–447.

Leonard C.M., Voeller, K.K.S., Lombardino, L.J., Morris, M.K., Hynd, G.W., Alexander, A.W., Andersen, H.G., Garofalakis, M., Honeyman, J.C., Mao, J., Agee, O.F. and Staab, E.V. (1993). Anomalous cerebral structure in dyslexia revealed with Magnetic Resonance Imaging. *Archives of Neurology, 50,* 461–469.

Levinson, H.N. (1990). The diagnostic value of cerebellar–vestibular tests in detecting learning disabilities, dyslexia and attention deficit disorder. *Perceptual and Motor Skills, 71,* 67–82.

Livingstone, M.S., Rosen, G.D., Drislane, F.W. and Galaburda, A.M. (1991). Physiological and anatomical evidence for a magnocellular deficit in developmental dyslexia. *Proceedings of the National Academy of Sciences of the USA, 88,* 7943–7947.

Lovegrove, W.J., Garzia, R.P. and Nicholson, S.B. (1990). Experimental evidence of a transient system deficit in specific reading disability. *Journal of the American Optometric Association, 61,* 137–146.

Miles, E. (1989). *The Bangor Dyslexia Teaching System.* London: Whurr.

Nicolson, R.I. (1993). The Cognitive Operations Multimedia Battery (COMB). *Technical Report LRG 93/14,* Department of Psychology, University of Sheffield.

Nicolson, R.I. and Fawcett, A.J. (1990). Automaticity: A new framework for dyslexia research. *Cognition, 35,* 159–182.

Nicolson, R.I. and Fawcett, A.J. (1994a). Reaction times and dyslexia. *Quarterly Journal of Experimental Psychology, Section A. 47A,* 1–16.

Nicolson, R.I. and Fawcett, A.J. (1994b). Skill, learning and dyslexia: A connectionist analysis. Submitted.

Nicolson, R.I., Fawcett, A.J. and Dean, P. (1994). Time estimation deficits in developmental dyslexia: Evidence for cerebellar dysfunction. Submitted.

Roland, P.E., Eriksson, L., Widen, L. and Stone-Elander, S. (1989). Changes in regional cerebral oxidative metabolism induced by tactile learning and recognition in man. *European Journal of Neuroscience, 1,* 3–17.

Rosner, J. and Simon, D.P. (1971). The auditory analysis test: An initial report. *Journal of Learning Disabilities, 4,* 384–392.

Seidenberg, M.S. (1993). Connectionist models and cognitive theory. *Psychological Science, 4,* 228–235.

Shaywitz, B., Shaywitz, S., Liberman, I., Fletcher, J., Shankweiler, D., Duncan, J., Katz, L., Liberman, A., Francis, D., Dreyer, L., Crain, S., Brady, S., Fowler, A., Kier, L., Rosenfield, N., Gore, J. and Makuch, R. (1991). Neurolinguistic and biologic mechanisms in dyslexia. In D.D. Duane and D.B. Gray (Eds.), *The Reading Brain: The biological basis of dyslexia.* Parkton, MD: York Press.

Siegel, L.S. (1989). IQ is irrelevant to the definition of learning disabilities. *Journal of Learning Disabilities, 22,* 469–479.

Stanovich, K.E. (1988). The right and wrong places to look for the cognitive locus of reading disability. *Annals of Dyslexia, 38,* 154–177.

Stanovich, K.E. (1991). Discrepancy definitions of reading disability: Has intelligence led us astray? *Reading Research Quarterly, 26,* 7–29

Tallal, P., Stark, R.E. and Mellits, D. (1985). The relationship between auditory temporal analysis and receptive language development: Evidence from studies of developmental language disorder. *Neuropsychologia, 23,* 527–534.

Thomson, M.E. (1984). *Developmental Dyslexia: Its nature, assessment and remediation.* London: Edward Arnold.

Vernon, P.A. (Ed.) (1987). *Speed of Information Processing and Intelligence.* Norwood, NJ: Ablex.

Wechsler, D. (1976). *Wechsler Intelligence Scale for Children Revised (WISC–R).* Slough, UK: NFER.

Author index

Subject index